Depression and Anxiety
in Later Life

A Johns Hopkins Press Health Book

■ ■ ■

Depression and Anxiety in Later Life

What Everyone Needs to Know

Mark D. Miller, M.D.
and Charles F. Reynolds III, M.D.

The Johns Hopkins University Press   Baltimore

Note to the reader: This book is not meant to substitute for medical care of people with depression or anxiety, and treatment should not be based solely on its contents. Instead, treatment must be developed in a dialogue between the individual and his or her physician. Our book has been written to help with that dialogue.

All efforts have been made to ensure the accuracy of the information contained in this book as of the date of publication. The authors and the publisher expressly disclaim responsibility for any adverse outcomes arising from the use or application of the information contained herein.

The authors and publisher have made reasonable efforts to determine that the selection and dosage of drugs, devices, and treatments discussed in this text conform to the practices of the general medical community. The drugs, devices, and treatments described do not necessarily have specific approval by the U.S. Food and Drug Administration for use as they are recommended. In view of ongoing research, changes in governmental regulations, and the constant flow of information relating to drug therapy and drug reactions, the reader is urged to check the package insert of each drug for any change in indications and dosage and for warnings and precautions. This is particularly important when the recommended agent is a new and/or an infrequently used drug.

© 2012 The Johns Hopkins University Press
All rights reserved. Published 2012
Printed in the United States of America on acid-free paper
9 8 7 6 5 4 3 2 1

The Johns Hopkins University Press
2715 North Charles Street
Baltimore, Maryland 21218-4363
www.press.jhu.edu

Library of Congress Cataloging-in-Publication Data

Miller, Mark D., 1955–
  Depression and anxiety in later life : what everyone needs to know / Mark D. Miller and Charles F. Reynolds III.
      p. cm. — (Johns Hopkins Press health book)
  Includes bibliographical references and index.
  ISBN 978-1-4214-0629-9 (hdbk. : alk. paper) — ISBN 978-1-4214-0630-5 (pbk. : alk. paper) — ISBN 978-1-4214-0707-4 (electronic) — ISBN 1-4214-0629-2 (hdbk. : alk. paper) — ISBN 1-4214-0630-6 (pbk. : alk. paper) — ISBN 1-4214-0707-8 (electronic)
  1. Depression in old age—Popular works. 2. Older people—Mental health—Popular works. 3. Older people—Health and hygiene—Popular works. 4. Aging—Popular works. I. Reynolds, Charles F., 1947– II. Title.
  RC537.5.M5385 2012
  618.97′68527—dc23   2012000021

A catalog record for this book is available from the British Library.

Special discounts are available for bulk purchases of this book. For more information, please contact Special Sales at 410-516-6936 or specialsales@press.jhu.edu.

CONTENTS

Thanks to numerous medical advances, humans are living longer, on average, than at any previous time in history. The average lifespan for American men is 77 years, and for American women, 80 years. By living longer, we have opportunities that weren't available to previous generations, but we also have a greater chance of accumulating chronic medical problems, experiencing various stresses that can lead to depression or anxiety, and developing memory impairment or dementia. Depression and anxiety disorders are two mental health issues that can burden up to half of older adults, some for the first time, others as a recurring challenge to their quality of life.

Contrary to the beliefs of many people, however, neither depression nor excessive anxiety is a normal part of aging. The risk factors for becoming depressed or excessively anxious are many and varied. They range from the grief of losing a loved one to the crushing disability of chronic pain to fears of running out of money.

Successful aging, on the other hand, requires that people adapt to the changing circumstances that accompany the process of getting older. People who can better control the risk factors stand a better chance of keeping depression and anxiety out of their lives as they age and, therefore, of enjoying the people and activities that bring them pleasure and fulfillment.

You may be reading this book as an older adult who senses or knows that something isn't quite right, as someone who has experienced depression or anxiety in the past and wants to make the most of an approaching retirement, or as the adult child of an older person. Our aim is to give you the latest knowledge about understanding depression and anxiety and their most common underlying risk factors for older adults.

We are two geriatric psychiatrists with over 50 years of combined experience treating older patients and conducting mental health research. This is our second book about mental health issues for older adults. We wrote our first, *Living Longer Depression Free*, about late-life depression and effective treatments. Since the release of that book in 2002, medical science has learned much more about risk factors for depression and for anxiety, which often occurs with depression.

This book provides information about recognizing, treating, and preventing these risks, which we frame around questions we frequently hear from our patients:

- I'm getting forgetful. Do I have dementia?
- How do I cope with my chronic illness or disability?
- What can be done about my chronic pain?
- Why do I feel so tired?
- How do I cope with the loss of my loved one?
- How can I stop or avoid overusing alcohol or prescription drugs?
- How do I achieve healthy body weight and good nutrition?
- How can I preserve or reactivate my sex life?
- How can I prepare for life's final phase?
- How do I make sense of my life and continue to lead a fulfilling life?

The struggle implied by each of these questions can lead a given person to feel anxious, demoralized, or depressed but also, we hope, motivated to learn more and take action.

In some instances, biological or chemical processes related to the factors alluded to in these questions can cause depression or anxiety. Conversely, having a rational discussion about each question and understanding treatment options can provide some relief and hope. Each of the chapters in part II of this book explores one of these questions to help you seek the best options for preventing or minimizing anxiety and depression as a result of that factor. Part I explains our current understanding of depression and anxiety and discusses the relationship between the two.

Whether you read the book from cover to cover or by selecting the chapters of most interest or relevance to you, we want to give you enough practical guidance to make informed choices either for yourself or for someone you're concerned about. Depression and excessive anxiety are *not* natural or inevitable parts of aging, and we hope that our explanations and suggestions will persuade you to make positive changes to keep depression and anxiety at bay.

Part I

Understanding Mood Disorders:
Knowledge Is Power

ONE

What You Need to Know about Depression

Most people experience the blues or feel low at some point in their lives, often after a stressful event, such as an illness or a loss. Sometimes the blues can show up for no apparent reason, which can be perplexing. When feelings of sadness, despair, or disinterest in normally pleasurable activities are short lived, lasting a few hours or a few days, people tend to shrug them off and move on. When these feelings last for more than two weeks and interfere with a person's ability to work or socialize, the "blues" have evolved into a medical illness called depression.

Depression is classified as a mood disorder, but it can involve both mood (psychological) and physical symptoms. Psychological symptoms can include the feelings already described as well as worsened concentration and guilty ruminations or even thoughts of death. When psychological symptoms are accompanied by symptoms of physical distress, such as sleep problems, appetite or weight changes, and lowered energy levels or motivation, the illness is termed major depression, or major depressive disorder. Like most afflictions, major depression can have mild, moderate, or severe effects on a given person's functioning.

Other forms of depression include

- minor depression, when a person has fewer symptoms than with major depression, and the symptoms are less severe, although they still interfere to some degree with everyday function
- dysthymia (from the Greek *dys-* meaning "bad" and *thymos* meaning "feeling or spirit"), which refers to chronic minor depression lasting for two years or more

- bipolar disorder, in which individuals have periodic mood swings between mania, or the less intense hypomania, and depression; hypomania and mania include a spectrum of symptoms—feeling "too good" (elation, having grandiose thoughts or plans), "too activated" (needing less sleep, having rapid thoughts or speech, being intensely active), and sometimes irritable
- psychotic depression, when depression causes individuals to lose their grasp on reality and harbor false beliefs or delusions; for example, a person with psychotic depression might say, "I know I am dying of cancer," when there is no medical evidence to suggest that the belief is true

Anybody can be afflicted with depression, no matter their age, ethnicity, social background, or success. In fact, many people who have achieved remarkable success in life have struggled with depression. To name only a few, Abraham Lincoln, sixteenth president of the United States; Buzz Aldrin, astronaut and second man to walk on the moon; Janet Jackson, singer and actress; and Amy Tan, author of *The Joy Luck Club* and other works, have all experienced major depression. Although anyone can become depressed, certain risk factors make it more likely for some people to develop the illness. Common risk factors in older people include medical illness, loss of a loved one, and isolation.

Among older adults, depression is a common problem. Of people older than age 60 who live in the community, 15 percent experience depressive symptoms that make it more difficult for them to function and lead a full life. For some of these people, depression is an illness they have not previously experienced, while others have had depressive episodes earlier in life as well. Depression is seen more frequently in older people who are medically ill (35% of those attending a medical clinic, and 50% of those in a hospital or diagnosed with cancer). Older people are less likely to report symptoms—which may include physical complaints like pain, constipation, low energy, and interrupted sleep—to their doctor, thinking that these problems are just a part of getting older. Also, these types of symptoms can be caused by various medical conditions as well as depression, which makes depression hard to recognize at times.

As for other illnesses, there are safe and effective treatments for depression, but regrettably, many people—older and younger alike—hesitate to seek help for depressive symptoms. Some people feel they should be able to handle the symptoms themselves. This thinking is inaccurate; people with serious depression can't simply "snap out of it," and without adequate treatment, the symptoms can continue for months or years and can become worse. Other people worry that depression is a sign of weakness or laziness. It isn't. Getting medical help can curb or eliminate the symptoms and enable the person to participate actively in life.

This chapter will help you recognize depression in yourself or another person, appreciate the risk factors for developing depression, and understand how the various treatment and management options work. We also give some information about lessening the chances of developing depression.

Recognizing Depression

Depression manifests in many different ways. Sometimes it can be easy to recognize, but other times, it's not so easy. Some of the physical symptoms, like changes in appetite or sleep, that can indicate depression in younger people are changes that older people experience as part of aging or because of a physical illness. Also, older people less frequently report emotional feelings to their doctor than younger people do.

The stories of Phyllis and Sam demonstrate two different faces of depression, the first hard for family members to miss, and the second hard to detect.

Phyllis, a 71-year-old retired bank teller, had never married but had always been involved with her close-knit family. She had two sisters and attended all the birthday and holiday celebrations with them and their families. Over several months, her sisters noticed that Phyllis was declining more and more invitations, often saying that her back or knee pain was flaring up again and she couldn't relieve it. One of her sisters offered to introduce her to her own doctor for a second opinion, but Phyllis refused the offer. Her other sister remarked that Phyllis seemed short-tempered and irritable on the phone. While visiting Phyllis at her

Table 1.1. Criteria for Major Depression

Criterion	Description
1. Depressed mood	Having a depressed mood most of the day and nearly every day; the patient may report his own mood, such as feeling sad or empty, or another person may observe and report the patient's mood, such as appearing tearful
2. Loss of interest in activities	Displaying markedly diminished interest or pleasure in all, or most, activities; this loss of interest occurs most of the day and nearly every day, reported by the patient or observed by others
3. Changes in body weight	Experiencing at least one of the following: ■ significant weight loss when not dieting ■ weight gain with an increase of more than 5% of body weight in one month ■ a decrease or increase in appetite nearly every day
4. Sleep issues	Being unable to sleep (insomnia) nearly every day, or being excessively sleepy or sleeping an excessive amount (hypersomnia) nearly every day
5. Physically overactive or underactive	Being physically restless or agitated nearly every day, or being physically weary and lethargic nearly every day; these symptoms are observed by other people and aren't just feelings reported by the patient
6. Diminished energy level	Feeling fatigued or experiencing a loss of energy nearly every day
7. Negative feelings about oneself	Having feelings of worthlessness nearly every day, or having feelings of excessive or inappropriate guilt nearly every day; the guilty feelings may be delusional or have no basis, and they are not merely self-reproach or guilt about being sick
8. Diminished mental ability	Experiencing a diminished ability to think or concentrate nearly every day, or displaying indecisiveness nearly every day; the patient may report changes in mental ability or others may observe them
9. Negative thoughts or actions	Any of the following symptoms: ■ having recurrent thoughts of death (not just a fear of dying) ■ entertaining the idea of suicide without a specific plan ■ making a suicide attempt or a specific plan for committing suicide

Source: Adapted from American Psychiatric Association, *Diagnostic and Statistical Manual of Mental Disorders*, 4th ed., DSM-IV-TR (2000), www.mental-health-today .com/dep/dsm.htm.

home, both sisters were surprised that her usually neat housekeeping had declined to the point where piles of unwashed laundry, dirty dishes, and unopened mail lay around the house. When Phyllis declined another invitation, saying she didn't know if she would still be around by then, her sisters decided together that Phyllis needed help for depression, and they insisted that she speak to her doctor.

Sam, age 80, had been a widower for 20 years, since his wife had died of cancer. They had enjoyed a good marriage, with two children, and now five grandchildren, all of whom lived in the same city. Sam's daughter, Amy, invited her father for dinner on most Sundays, and often the whole family gathered for cookouts in the summertime. Sam still played golf twice a week with some old friends from his former days as a management consultant for a large corporation. He suffered from chronic back pain and had had two back surgeries for bulging discs, but he was not the type to complain. During his business career, he had learned to maintain a cheery disposition, and he tried hard to continue being cheerful despite his back pain, to "keep up appearances," as he told his doctor. When his doctor asked about his week, Sam described it as "a series of obligations that I get through and then try to sleep." Sam also revealed that he had trouble relaxing enough to go to sleep without a glass or two of red wine, and occasionally, when he woke in the night and couldn't get back to sleep, he tried a glass of scotch.

Phyllis was clearly irritable, becoming socially isolated, and having difficulty functioning with daily tasks, all commonly seen with depression. Her offhand remark indicating a pessimistic view of her future finally spurred her sisters to act and get her professional help. Sam, on the other hand, was a pretty good actor, who maintained his "obligations," as he called them, and didn't complain, so his children and friends suspected nothing. However, his candor with his physician about his chronic pain, difficulty staying cheerful, and self-medication with alcohol meant that he finally did get the treatment he needed for depression.

Mental health professionals use nine criteria, listed in table 1.1, to evaluate an individual for possible depression. A diagnosis of major depression is made if a person displays five or more of the nine criteria during a two-week period and hadn't previously had that set of symptoms. Also, at least one of the first two criteria in the list—depressed mood and loss of interest in activities—must be part of the person's

Table 1.2. The Patient Health Questionnaire–9 (PHQ-9) for Depression

Over the last two weeks, how often have you been bothered by any of the following problems?	Not at all	Several days	More than half the days	Nearly every day
1. Little interest or pleasure in doing things	0	1	2	3
2. Feeling down, depressed, or hopeless	0	1	2	3
3. Trouble falling or staying asleep, or sleeping too much	0	1	2	3
4. Feeling tired or having little energy	0	1	2	3
5. Poor appetite or overeating	0	1	2	3
6. Feeling bad about yourself, that you are a failure, or that you have let yourself or your family down	0	1	2	3
7. Trouble concentrating on things, such as reading the newspaper or watching TV	0	1	2	3
8. Moving or speaking noticeably slowly, or the opposite—being so fidgety or restless that you have been moving around more than usual	0	1	2	3
9. Thoughts that you would be better off dead or of hurting yourself in some way	0	1	2	3
Add the columns:				
Add the totals of each column for a total score:				

symptoms for a diagnosis of major depression. A diagnosis of minor depression is made when a person has only three symptoms, with one being either depressed mood or a loss of interest in activities.

Screening Questionnaires

You may have visited your primary care physician in the past and filled out a survey or questionnaire asking about your mood, thoughts, and feelings. Many physicians use this type of tool to screen individuals for depression because it helps identify the collection of symptoms

	Not difficult at all	Somewhat difficult	Very difficult	Extremely difficult
10. If you checked off *any* problem on this questionnaire so far, how *difficult* have these problems made it for you to do your work, take care of things at home, or get along with other people?				

SCORING INFORMATION:
A person may have major depression if:

a. Item 1 or item 2 has been circled as "more than half the days" or "nearly every day," *and*
b. at least four additional items have been circled as "more than half the days" or "nearly every day."

A person may have another depressive condition if:

a. Item 1 or item 2 has been circled as "more than half the days" or "nearly every day," and
b. one to three additional items have been circled as "more than half the days" or "nearly every day."

The severity of depression is indicated by the total score calculated from the questionnaire responses, as follows:

Total Score	Severity
1–4	Minor depression
5–9	Mild major depression
10–14	Moderate major depression
15–19	Moderately severe major depression
20–27	Severe depression

Source: The PHQ-9 was developed by Drs. Robert L. Spitzer, Janet B. W. Williams, Kurt Kroenke, and colleagues, with an educational grant from Pfizer, Inc.

(called a syndrome) that adds up to a diagnosis of depression. It can be easy for a physician to focus on one symptom or area and not make the connection between seemingly disparate symptoms during a short office visit. The questionnaire uses a rating scale that describes a diagnosis of depression in a more objective way than as a collection of subjective feelings or thoughts. These survey tools can also be used to estimate the severity of depression and track progress in recovering from depression over time.

Individuals can also use these screening tools to perform a self-assessment of their mood. One commonly used screening tool for depression is reprinted in table 1.2, along with instructions for scoring and interpreting the questionnaire. When you fill out this or a similar questionnaire, whether at home or at your physician's office, fill it out honestly. Try to put aside any feelings of embarrassment or thoughts that you are displaying weakness by admitting how you feel, think, and act. You have nothing to gain from not being true to yourself, and everything to gain from receiving an accurate diagnosis and appropriate treatment.

Because a diagnosis of major depression is formed from a collection of several symptoms, focusing on just one or two symptoms might not trigger you to consider depression as a possible cause of them. Older individuals in particular commonly attribute individual symptoms to the process of aging. When all symptoms are examined together, however, they can point to depression. This is why the survey tools can be particularly useful, both for helping a patient understand the connections between seemingly unrelated symptoms and for helping a doctor "build a case" and persuade the individual to seek treatment to feel better.

Risk Factors for Developing Depression

An individual's risk of developing depression can depend on a huge range of factors. Some common risk factors for depression, particularly in older individuals, are

- medical illness or disability that robs a person of his ability to carry on as usual or that undermines his independence
- impaired brain function (cognition) and dementia
- stress from struggling with a punitive or capricious boss, a dysfunctional marriage, or children with illness, addictions, or behavioral problems
- social isolation and loneliness
- grief over the death of a loved one

Other, less obvious, risks are being female or having an over- or underactive thyroid gland, vitamin B12 deficiency, or small strokes (of which the person may not even be aware). Table 1.3 summarizes these and other risk factors for developing depression. Those that are particular risks for older people are described in more detail in later chapters of this book. Some of the factors in table 1.3 are not necessarily of greater risk for older individuals, although they may contribute to an older person's depression, so we discuss them briefly in the following pages.

Family History

At a doctor visit, your physician may ask whether any of your close relatives—your grandparents, parents, siblings, or children—have been diagnosed with depression in the past. The reason for this is that family history, or genetics, can be a strong risk factor for developing depression. Studies of identical twins, even those reared apart, have shown strikingly similar rates of depression in each twin, which suggests that their shared genetics gives them similar vulnerability to depression, despite their environment. Researchers have also shown that people with a greater number of relatives with depression stand a greater chance of having inherited that risk for depression.

The genetic risk for depression can skip a generation, however. Parents who both have depression will not necessarily have children who develop depression, but it might show up again in a subsequent generation. Most researchers believe that mood disorders result from a culmination of factors, of which genetic vulnerability is just one. Anyone can become depressed if enough risk factors accumulate, but for a person who inherits a genetic vulnerability, fewer additional risk factors can bring on major depression. Individuals with a strong genetic vulnerability don't necessarily need other risk factors to become severely depressed. People with this vulnerability will sometimes say they are confused by how badly they feel, because they cannot point to a particular event or malady in their lives on which to blame the depression.

Bipolar disorder is known to be inherited in families, and research has even identified specific genes that transmit the risk. Bipolar disorder, also called manic depression, refers to a pattern of abnormal moods that can swing either too high or too low. The high swings are known as mania and are characterized by a period of at least several days of feeling euphoric or irritable, with accompanying symptoms such as less need for sleep, rapidly shifting thoughts or speech, grandiose plans or actions, inflated self-importance, increased sex drive, and the tendency to spend too much money or engage in other risky

Table 1.3. Risk Factors for Developing Depression

Risk factor	Description	Chapter(s) with details
Female gender	Women may be at greater risk because of female hormone cycles or the lack of them in menopause, as well as often bearing a disproportionate burden of family responsibilities.	10
Family history	Some people inherit a vulnerability to developing depression. It may take fewer risk factors, and sometimes no other risk factors, for depression to develop.	1
Past history of depression	One prior episode increases the risk of another one. Depression, in general, is a chronic (long-term) condition.	1
Current depressive symptoms	Having some symptoms of depression is a risk for developing the full syndrome of major depression.	1
Personality traits and disorders	Personality traits are a person's characteristic attitudes and actions. Someone with a tendency to be very dependent on others may fall into a panic or state of depression if the person he depends on most goes away. A personality disorder occurs when the sum of personality traits interferes with a person maintaining satisfying give-and-take relationships.	1
Seasonal mood change	During the dark, short days of winter, some individuals feel leaden, lack energy, spend a great deal of time in bed but awake feeling unrested, become socially isolated, crave carbohydrates, and gain weight. These symptoms can be caused by seasonal affective disorder (SAD), which typically eases in the spring and summer months, only to return again the next fall or winter.	1
Anxiety disorder	Being anxious too often or too severely tends to limit activity and can become demoralizing or depressing.	2
Medical condition	Some illnesses cause depression by altering the chemical balance in the brain or by affecting brain function, while other illnesses result in physical limitations that lead to depression.	3, 4
Disability	Physical or mental limitations on function can lead to demoralization and depression.	3, 4
Chronic pain	It is depressing to have chronic pain, particularly if it limits activities, interferes with sleep, or is unrelenting with treatment.	5

Chronic insomnia	A good night's sleep is restorative and a protective factor from depression. Poor sleep robs one of energy, stamina, and concentration and increases the risk for depression.	6
Caregiver	Caregiving may be a labor of love, but it can become a strain over time and lead to exhaustion, demoralization, and depression, sometimes complicated by self-medication with alcohol or drugs.	3, 4, 10
Bereavement	Losing a loved one can bring on depression even months after the death.	7
Living alone	Having little or no companionship or social support is a risk for depression.	throughout
Divorced	Married individuals show less depression. The stress of a divorce can bring on depression.	throughout
Widowed	Losing a spouse has multiple implications in addition to bereavement, such as needing to assume new roles to take over tasks and responsibilities that the late spouse handled.	7, 10
Alcohol or drug abuse	Alcohol and some drugs slow down the flow of nerve impulses within the brain, contributing to depression and making it worse. Furthermore, excess drinking or illicit drug use frequently leads to personal crises like job loss, divorce, injury, or illness, which can trigger depression.	8
Living with an addict (alcohol, drug, gambling)	The unpredictability of an addicted individual's behavior and the tension between complicity and confrontation can contribute to relatives of the addict feeling trapped, hopeless, and depressed.	8
Obesity	In addition to being associated with self-consciousness or low self-esteem, obesity can limit activity, interfere with job performance, impair sleep, and increase the risk for high blood pressure, diabetes, and heart disease, all of which can contribute to depression.	9
Emotional distress	Distress that leads to depression can stem from family, work, marital, or financial concerns, as well as from worry about living arrangements, such as the need for a care facility.	10, 11, 12

behaviors. The low swings are a decline from normal mood to a state of depression that is identical to major depression. Bipolar disorder, the details of which can easily fill a book of its own, usually requires management from mental health professionals. For interested readers, some references are included in the resources.

Personality Traits

Personality traits, or temperament, are behavior patterns and ways of thinking about and perceiving the world that are formed early in childhood and remain more or less stable throughout one's life. Certain personality traits can predispose a person to developing depression. For example, some babies have an anxious temperament and require lots of comforting and reassurance right from birth. If the parent can meet the demands, then there is a good match. On the other hand, if the child's demands are too high or the parent's ability to meet them is more limited, then the child grows up in a state of constant distress. This distress can affect the quality of all subsequent relationships (peers, friends, coworkers, spouses), putting the individual at risk of depression. Completing the circle, a particularly demanding child can increase a parent's stress levels, which may lead to depression and place further limitations on the parent's ability to nurture the child.

Researchers categorize personality traits as, for example, shy versus outgoing and predominantly "thinking" versus "feeling." People with personality traits that interfere with their ability to function in social or workplace settings are said to have a personality disorder. Mental health professionals distinguish ten personality disorders, and some of them are risk factors for developing depression. For example, individuals with dependent personality disorder have an inordinate need to be helped or comforted by others and often become dependent on others for even basic functions. If the person on whom they depend dies or leaves, they are thrown into a state of panic or depression.

Seasonal Mood Change

The weather can also affect mood. Winter blues, also known as seasonal affective disorder (SAD), causes susceptible individuals to feel that their energy level and mood sink with the gradually shortening and darkening days as winter approaches. These people describe feeling "leaden" and lacking energy, sex drive, motivation, and the desire to socialize. They have a hard time rising in the morning, have no desire to be active, and crave carbohydrate-laden foods, resulting in weight gain. They feel weepy and miserable and that they must push themselves to complete even mundane tasks. Spouses and friends of a person with SAD can feel frustrated or angry with his tendency to avoid socializing or participating in recreational activities.

The phenomenon of SAD is most common in people living at more northerly latitudes of the northern hemisphere and in people originally from a region closer to the equator but now living farther north. Other individuals at risk of SAD are shift workers who see little daylight, those who live or work in windowless buildings, those who keep their drapes pulled shut all day, and those who have cataracts (the cloudiness of the eye lens restricts the amount of light reaching the retina). The mechanism of SAD involves biological rhythms that are not adjusted as they should be by available sunlight.

The Long-Term Complications of Depression

Sometimes, people with major depression will get better on their own, without treatment. The chance of a spontaneous recovery is unpredictable, however, and in the meantime, months or even years can go by. Untreated depression can persist for a decade or longer, and if it is severe enough, can result in the afflicted person dying. Death can result from suicide (severely depressed people have an increased risk for completed suicide), neglected health care, attempts to self-medicate with risky behaviors such as alcohol or drug abuse, or accidents caused by impaired judgment while in a state of depression, including accidental overdose of prescribed medication. Untreated major depression also increases the risk of complications after surgery, because it slows the healing process and increases the risk of dying from heart disease or cancer. The good news, however, is that adequately treating depression can eliminate the risk of these negative long-term consequences.

Specific Risks for Suicide

Individuals with severe major depression may have passive thoughts about welcoming death or may think about actually taking their own life. The combination of depression and intense anxiety increases the risk of following through on suicidal thoughts, especially when sleep deprivation is also a factor. Alcohol or drug use can also increase the chance of a person trying to follow through, because alcohol and drugs numb their inhibition. Women tend to make more attempts at suicide, but men usually use more lethal methods and are therefore more likely to complete the act. Older individuals talk less about their suicidal thoughts than younger people, decreasing the chance for detection and intervention, and when they make up their mind, older individuals follow through more often. Over the entire population, those with the highest risk of completed suicide are older, white, recently widowed men who consume alcohol.

Getting Treatment for Depression

Several treatments are available for depression, with antidepressant medications and psychotherapy, or talk therapy, being the two most commonly used. Other treatments include electroconvulsive and stimulation therapies.

One important aspect of treatment is for patients and families to learn more about depression and how to improve the chances of successful treatment. In addition to following instructions for the selected approach, patients and families should have realistic goals for recovery. Depression treatments can take time to work, and the improvements are likely to be gradual. Sometimes, family members or close friends will notice a change for the better before the depressed person does.

Medications

Antidepressant medications are the current cornerstone of modern treatment for severe depression. In many cases, the exact mechanisms by which these drugs relieve depression are unclear, but the prevailing theory is that antidepressants increase the availability of certain chemical messengers in the brain. These chemical messengers, called neurotransmitters, include seratonin, norepinephrine, and dopamine.

One perplexing mystery is why a given drug alleviates depression in one person and not in another. In fact, any given antidepressant medication is effective in achieving a complete remission of depressive symptoms in only about half of patients who get an adequate trial of the drug (at least four weeks at an appropriate dose). A growing theme in medicine today is the concept of personalized medicine, where doctors use information about an individual's risk factors, ethnicity, and genetic makeup (if available) to try to predict which treatment will work best for that person. The emerging field of pharmacogenomics involves identifying specific genes that affect how a person will respond to a particular medication. As the techniques are refined, genetic subtyping will likely become more common and will lead to better treatment outcomes.

A variety of antidepressant medications are available, as shown in table 1.4. The factors a doctor uses to select which medication is most appropriate for a person with depression include age, frailty, concurrent medical problems and other medications, insomnia, agitation, psychosis, and concurrent anxiety. The goal is to choose a drug that might also benefit or at least not exacerbate these other conditions.

Every drug has its side effects, and antidepressants are no exception. Typically, the class of drugs called SSRIs (selective serotonin reuptake inhibitors) cause the fewest side effects. Some people won't experience any, or will have only a few, side effects, and they may go away within a few days or weeks of taking the medication. Every person is different, however, so it's particularly important to report all possible side effects to your doctor. In general, if you cannot tolerate the side effects while taking one class of antidepressant medication, your doctor can try another drug that may work just as well to relieve the depression but has fewer side effects. Sometimes, adjusting the dose or changing the time of day when the medication is taken can reduce them. Also, some medications that you take for other conditions may interact with certain antidepressants with dangerous effects. Be certain to give your doctor a list of all medications that you take, including over-the-counter medications.

When you are first prescribed an antidepressant medication, your doctor will closely track your progress and tolerance of the medication. You can expect to see your doctor every one to three weeks, depending on the severity of your symptoms and speed of progress.

Table 1.4. Commonly Prescribed Antidepressant Medications and Possible Side Effects

Drug category	Examples (brand names in parentheses)	Possible side effects
Selective serotonin reuptake inhibitors, or SSRIs	fluoxetine (Prozac), citalopram (Celexa), sertraline (Zoloft), paroxetine (Paxil), escitalopram (Lexapro)	■ Headache (usually goes away within a few days) ■ Nausea (usually goes away within a few days) ■ Sleeplessness or drowsiness (usually goes away after the first few weeks) ■ Agitation ■ Sexual problems (such as reduced sex drive; problems having and enjoying sex)
Serotonin and norepinephrine reuptake inhibitors, or SNRIs	venlafaxine (Effexor), duloxetine (Cymbalta)	Same as above
Tricyclics	nortriptyline (Pamelor, Aventyl), amitriptyline (Elavil), imipramine (Tofranil), desipramine (Norpramin)	■ Dry mouth ■ Constipation ■ Bladder problems (difficulty emptying the bladder; urine stream not as strong as usual) ■ Sexual problems (such as reduced sex drive; problems having and enjoying sex) ■ Blurred vision (usually goes away quickly) ■ Drowsiness
Tetracyclics	trazodone (Desyrel), maprotiline (Ludiomil)	Sedation, weight gain, dry mouth
Monoamine oxidase inhibitors, or MAOIs	phenelzine (Nardil), tranylcypromine (Parnate)	Combined with foods and medicines containing high levels of the chemical tyramine can cause a sharp increase in blood pressure, which can then cause a stroke; tyramine is found in some cheeses, wines, and pickles and in some medications, including decongestants and over-the-counter cold medicine (Pharmacists distribute complete lists of foods and other drugs that must be monitored or avoided when taking MAOIs.)

Source: National Institute of Mental Health, *Mental Health Medications*, NIH Publication No. 08-3929. Revised in 2008.

As the person receiving treatment, your responsibilities are to follow through with the doctor's recommendations for taking the medication and to give regular reports about the medication's effects. Never change the dose or stop taking the medication before speaking with your doctor. Last, try to be patient: it often takes as long as four to six weeks for an antidepressant medication to provide significant relief of depression, with further improvements over an additional four weeks. Common early signs of improvement are sleeping better, being less anxious, and having a better appetite, followed by having greater energy. Mood and libido (sexual drive) are typically the last things to improve.

Sometimes, for reasons not well understood, antidepressants can stop working after being effective for one or more years. In these cases, a dose increase might restore a normal mood, but sometimes another treatment is required.

COMMON MYTHS ABOUT ANTIDEPRESSANT MEDICATIONS

We counter the following myths and misinformation with facts so that people with depression can be open minded and willing to seek treatment that will help them.

1. Antidepressants will cause me to be suicidal. Whether antidepressants increase suicidal tendencies has, understandably, generated a lot of public interest, and it has also been closely examined in scientific studies. The Food and Drug Administration (FDA) currently has a warning in place for the use of these drugs with children, adolescents, and young adults up to age 25, but not for people older than 25.

Because an antidepressant medication can take weeks to provide significant improvement in depressive symptoms, it's entirely possible for a depressed person with suicidal impulses to act on those impulses after starting an antidepressant, before it has had a chance to improve the depressive symptoms. In a person with depression, the levels of chemical neurotransmitters in the brain can also fluctuate daily, like the ebb and flow of other phenomena in nature, such as ocean tides, which means that depressive symptoms continue to fluctuate during the early stage of treatment with antidepressants. Thus, depressive symptoms, including suicidal thoughts, can worsen even after the individual begins taking an antidepressant. For this reason, the FDA also recommends that patients with suicidal thoughts be seen by their doctor more frequently and watched more carefully in the early stages of treatment until it is certain that they are on the road to recovery.

2. Antidepressants are like antibiotics. Antibiotics (when prescribed correctly) treat bacterial infections. For many relatively common bacterial infections, like strep throat, antibiotics are prescribed for a short period (only one or two weeks). Once the patient has taken the full antibiotic course, the infection and its symptoms are usually gone. Antidepressants do not work in this way. They do not instantly relieve the low mood, lack of energy, or sleep disturbance that can result from depression. Rather, they work gradually, often taking four to six weeks to take full effect.

Unlike antibiotics, whose sole job is to kill unwanted bacteria, antidepressant medications attempt to correct chemical imbalances related to the depression. Antidepressants are more like insulin, which a person with diabetes must take every day. They work to reestablish a balance, or synchrony, in complex neurological systems that have gone awry. It takes time, therefore, for the effect to take place and be noticeable. Sometimes, antidepressants need to be taken for the long term, even for a lifetime, to keep serious bouts of depression from returning.

3. Antidepressants are like pain relievers. Pain relievers for headaches and muscle aches are typically taken as needed. Antidepressant medications don't work in this way. They are not designed to be taken only when someone is having a bad day and feels depressed. For antidepressants to relieve depressive symptoms, they must be taken daily for extended periods.

4. Antidepressants are addictive drugs. Antidepressants are not addictive, and they don't produce a "high," or state of euphoria. The decision to use antidepressant medications for the long term is an informed choice made by individuals in consultation with their doctor. The reason to continue taking antidepressants is to seek long-term relief from depression; doing so does not equate to the person having an addictive condition.

Some antidepressant drugs, if stopped too abruptly, can cause withdrawal, such as flu-like symptoms, muscle aches, nightmares, or muscle twitches. These symptoms can be avoided by slowly tapering the daily dose of the drug over several weeks when the decision is made to stop taking the medication.

5. *Antidepressants will make me feel drugged or like a zombie.* Like any medication, antidepressants have side effects, one of which can be sedation (drowsiness). Some antidepressants are more sedating than others. Some sedation can be a good thing for a depressed person with severe insomnia but not for one who is already sleeping too much. Sometimes, changing the medication dose, time of day when the medication is taken, or even switching to a different antidepressant may be options for alleviating sedation or other intolerable side effects.

6. *As soon as I begin to feel better, I won't need to take antidepressants anymore.* Many people whose depression is treated successfully with antidepressants feel confident that they can stop taking the medication when they no longer feel depressed. Our research has shown, however, that doing so is fraught with risk for a relapse into depression, because depressive illnesses are prone to recur. Studies of depression suggest that, to minimize the chance of depression recurring, an individual should take an antidepressant for six to nine months for the first episode, one to two years for the second episode, and a lifetime for the third or subsequent episode.

If your doctor has prescribed antidepressants, continue to take them as instructed until you jointly make the decision to stop them. Your doctor will give you advice on the best way to stop taking them to minimize withdrawal symptoms.

7. *Antidepressant medications will change my personality.* Antidepressants do not alter personality, but some antidepressants can cause subtle changes in the way a person feels. These changes are hopefully signs that the medication is working to relieve the person's depression. Sometimes, the SSRI medications can induce unwanted changes in emotions. Some patients complain of feeling emotionally blunted or unable to cry when they think they should be able to, and others say that they can't generate their usual creative impulses. These complaints can be addressed with dose adjustments or a switch to a different medication. It is important to be frank in reporting all medication effects to the doctor who prescribed the medication in order to minimize or eliminate these kinds of side effects.

Psychotherapy

The Austrian neurologist Sigmund Freud treated his patients with the "talking cure," which we now call psychotherapy. Unlike talking to a friend, hairdresser, or bartender, all of whom may be good listeners, a professionally trained psychotherapist understands mental illnesses such as depression and anxiety. The therapist uses both knowledge and experience to help individuals see their predicament or problem clearly, to view it from multiple angles, and to weigh options for change. The goal is to bring relief from the depression and anxiety symptoms and to help people search for and find fulfillment in life. The best way to understand how psychotherapy works may be to read a case study.

> Mildred, age 62, worked for a manufacturing company. Bill, her husband of 33 years, had died of a sudden heart attack nine months earlier, and though she had returned to work, she couldn't seem to stop bursting into tears when something reminded her of Bill. Since her work involved customer relations, her boss said that she had to get some help or take more time off, because he couldn't have her continuing to be emotionally unstable at work. Mildred was also having trouble sleeping and cried for hours alone at night. Her primary care doctor gave her a sleeping pill and an antidepressant. She slept better, but the medication didn't seem to stop her from feeling so sad or from crying so much.
>
> Mildred agreed that she needed more help, because she didn't know how to find relief for her awful feelings. On her first visit to a psychotherapist, she described how she stayed at home every night and on weekends, no longer attended church, and refused invitations from family and friends to venture out. When asked about Bill, she described him glowingly as a great father, husband, and companion. Her first husband had walked out, leaving her with three small children, whom she had raised alone until she remarried four years later. Mildred cried heavily when she recounted the plans that she and Bill had made to travel when they retired in a few short years. She felt she had been robbed and had lost her soul mate.
>
> Over the next three visits, Mildred talked at length about Bill's good attributes and how much she missed him. Her therapist listened carefully and encouraged her to keep talking to get a full picture of their

relationship. At the fourth visit, something shifted. Mildred began to talk about how Bill had sometimes frustrated her. Her therapist gently encouraged her to explain why. Mildred described Bill as having had a stubborn streak and said that they had argued often about him going to the doctor; Mildred never won those arguments. Bill hated going to doctors and prided himself for not taking any medications whatsoever, not even vitamins. He always said he felt "as strong as a horse," and indeed, he could carry a 50-pound bag of lawn fertilizer by himself and make it look easy, despite being 30 pounds overweight.

Bill had been wrong about his health, however; their neighbor found him unconscious beside the woodpile, where he had been splitting logs for the fireplace. The paramedics pronounced him dead at the scene, and an autopsy showed extensive coronary artery disease. He had died of a massive heart attack when a clot formed in one of the narrowed arteries that fed his heart muscle. Mildred tearfully described her thoughts and memories from the moment she got the call at work and knew immediately from the tone of her neighbor's voice that something terrible had happened. She seemed exhausted from recounting this story but also relieved to have a sympathetic ear to describe the way she had experienced her husband's death.

Mildred said she felt guilty and responsible for Bill's death, so her therapist asked her to explain how she had arrived at that conclusion. Mildred explained that it was her duty as his devoted wife to persuade him to get routine medical care, and that she should have tried harder and not given up when he'd stubbornly refused, especially since she now knew that he'd had undiagnosed heart disease. Her therapist reminded Mildred that she had, in fact, tried on several occasions to convince Bill to visit a doctor, and since he had not complained of chest pain, there hadn't been any particular cause for alarm. Her therapist was sympathetic and said she understood Mildred's wish to have been at his side when he died and her hope that he had not suffered for long.

When asked to describe all the tasks and chores that she now faced without Bill's help, Mildred produced a long list of what she had to learn to manage on her own, such as mowing the lawn, dealing with car repairs, and paying bills. What she missed the most, however, was the chance to travel when they were both retired. Mildred felt that she had been robbed of this dream, but she quickly stopped herself and added that she had no right to complain, since Bill was now dead, and her unfulfilled wish to travel seemed trivial in comparison. Her therapist pointed out that it is legitimate to acknowledge one's own needs, and that guilty feelings are common among survivors. The therapist continued by saying that Mildred's annoyance and even anger toward Bill for his complacency about medical care was completely within the range of normal feelings among people grieving the loss of a loved one.

With gentle encouragement along these lines, Mildred began to sleep better and stopped crying at work. She resumed going to church and accepted invitations to go out for dinner with family. When Mildred and her therapist agreed to stop their sessions after meeting for 12 consecutive weeks, Mildred summed up her current thoughts and feelings for Bill, saying that he was a good man whom she missed very much but also a stubborn man who bore some responsibility for his own death by refusing medical checkups that might have prolonged his life. She further acknowledged being angry with him for being inconsiderate of her needs and her future by not taking better care of himself. She also said that she felt angry with him for ruining her dream of traveling together in retirement and for saddling her with all the household responsibilities they had once shared. It wasn't easy for Mildred to admit her anger toward Bill, but her therapist's compassion and patience had allowed her to mourn while recognizing that Bill had flaws as well as admirable attributes.

After Mildred "owned" her feelings about Bill, both positive and negative, she could more easily let him rest in peace with a strong but gradually lightening sadness. The psychotherapist had helped Mildred to untangle her complicated emotions surrounding the sudden death of her husband and to acknowledge that her guilty feelings stemmed from trying to avoid her negative emotions about being "angry at a dead man," which had seemed absurd at first. Once Mildred acknowledged her need to look out for herself, her thoughts and feelings made more sense to her, and she could accept Bill's character and his death, while turning her attention to continuing to lead her own life.

There are several different types of psychotherapy that encompass various approaches and philosophies. Some types cover the entire spectrum of one's life while others target more specific areas.

PSYCHODYNAMIC THERAPY

Psychodynamic therapy focuses on a person's feelings in the present while maintaining an alertness for relevant connections from life experiences in the past. Individuals generally meet with their therapist for a 50-minute session once or twice per week, with the sessions continuing for several months to years. Each session focuses on their activities, thoughts, feelings, and dreams since the previous visit, as well as dreams and thoughts that link to prior life events. Therapists listen carefully for thoughts that are stimulated by or associated with the topic at hand and that may be a window into their patients' unconscious minds. Therapists make interpretations and links to early life experiences to help individuals develop insight and understand themselves better. Achieving insight is not always sufficient for a person to feel better, but it is the initial goal from which to continue exploring options for change that may bring more personal fulfillment.

INTERPERSONAL PSYCHOTHERAPY

Interpersonal psychotherapy, or IPT, focuses on how people interact with family, friends, coworkers, and any other significant person in their current lives. Rather than exploring early life experiences, as in psychodynamic therapy, IPT focuses on the present to reduce depressive symptoms. Individuals meet with a therapist once a week for only 12 to 16 weeks. This short duration provides an incentive to work on one focus, which is negotiated between therapists and participants, and to make progress before time runs out. The four foci that IPT targets are prolonged grief, role transition (to retirement, for example), role dispute (interpersonal conflict with a spouse, adult child, or boss, for example), and interpersonal role sensitivity or deficit (chronic problems in getting along with others).

Therapists help people explore the pros and cons of making various changes in the way they communicate, make decisions, or seek social connections, with the goal of reducing or eliminating the symptoms of depression. Early on in the treatment, depressed individuals are given the role of being "sick" to help relieve guilt and allow them space from their usual responsibilities until they begin to feel better.

IPT is often used along with antidepressants. Persons who do not have substantial improvement in their depressive symptoms after

16 weeks should try other therapies. A long-term form of IPT, with monthly sessions, can help maintain the gains achieved in the initial 12 to 16 sessions and is particularly suited to helping people with frequent role disputes to maintain their new (better) ways of coping.

COGNITIVE BEHAVIOR THERAPY

Cognitive behavior therapy, or CBT, helps individuals identify and alter automatic negative thoughts or ideas that they have about themselves or other people. They are given homework assignments to challenge their assumptions, be more proactive, and explore the possibility of new friends and activities. The goal is to make their lives more fulfilling and therefore leave them with fewer reasons to be depressed.

For example, someone who is invited to a party but doesn't want to go because he doesn't know any of the other guests and assumes that no one will like him is having an automatic negative thought. A CBT therapist would challenge this person to show evidence that his assumption is correct, and if he can't, the therapist points out the flaw in his logic and challenges him to test it by going to the party. The person's "homework" when he meets new people at the party is to see if he can identify dislike from the new people's attitudes or statements. What he might learn is that his assumptions actually keep him at an unfriendly distance from others, and that if he instead musters his courage to try a more forward, engaging approach, he might find that other people respond warmly to him in return.

This type of homework assignment helps the individual challenge automatic negative thoughts and realize that they are unsubstantiated. Testing new ways of doing things to bring about positive results is the next step toward feeling more optimistic and less depressed.

PROBLEM-SOLVING THERAPY FOR PRIMARY CARE

Problem-solving therapy for primary care (PST-PC) developed from CBT as a highly specific strategy to reverse the demoralization and low motivation that often characterize depression in later life. PST-PC is a short-term treatment with six to eight half-hour sessions that focuses on solving one pragmatic problem at a time.

The depressed individuals select the problems to address from a list that they generate, with the guidance of their therapist. After brainstorming possible solutions to the problem, individuals choose one solution and agree to a highly specific sequence of steps, which the therapist writes down for them to take home and implement. At their next meeting, they review successes or failures and then initiate a new round of problem solving. This cycle repeats for the duration of the six to eight meetings.

With a series of successes at problem solving, individuals' confidence builds and their feelings of helplessness and hopelessness wane. Even after the PST-PC therapy ends, the hoped-for goal is that the strategies learned during the sessions can be generalized and applied to other problems without the therapist's help. Periodic "booster" sessions with the therapist can also help individuals consolidate and apply the problem-solving strategies that they learned.

GROUP THERAPY

Depression affects not only people with the illness but also those around them. It can be depressing to live with an overly negative person who is irritable or has little interest in activities. The damage that depression can cause to relationships often requires some help to repair. For this reason, a psychotherapist may suggest that people with depression attend therapy sessions in a group with other people dealing with depression, or with their spouses or partners, or as a family. Group therapy can be an adaptation of one of the above therapies, led by a therapist and sometimes a co-therapist, but more often, it targets a specific problem area, such as grief, coping with a cancer diagnosis, living with a family member with dementia, or seeking support to resist an addictive behavior. Alcoholics Anonymous is an example of an organization that provides group therapy.

PRACTICAL TIPS

Some therapists are capable of providing more than one type of therapy to a given person, but most therapists offer only one type. Finding a good match between your needs and what a particular psychotherapist offers is sometimes an exercise in trial and error. Getting a recommendation from a friend or family member who has had a positive experience can work well for finding a therapist. You can also find a psychotherapist or psychiatrist who offers the type of therapy you're looking for by consulting your primary care physician, a local professional society (such as the American Psychological Association), or a yellow pages directory of local practitioners. Remember that the therapist is working for you, and therefore, it is entirely appropriate to ask about the person's philosophy and education and to interview more than one therapist before you decide with whom you wish to work.

If you decide to go to a psychotherapist, you can do several things to ensure the therapy is as effective as possible. Attend all appointments and participate actively. Psychotherapy takes time and multiple sessions to begin alleviating symptoms of depression. Although psychotherapy can take several months longer than antidepressants before you see the effects, there is some evidence that successful psychotherapy has a longer-lasting effect. If you have trouble with your psychotherapist's approach, or you're unsure of the usefulness of the sessions, then let the therapist know, but don't simply stop going to sessions. If after giving your therapist an adequate trial, you still don't feel you are making any progress, it may be worthwhile to try a different approach or even a different therapist.

Your therapist will help you establish some goals; here are a few that you may be encouraged to do.

- Keep a journal to note down both stressful and positive events, and review it.
- Make time every day for recreational and other activities that you enjoy.
- Think about positive outcomes for situations that occur in your day.
- Practice speaking up for yourself and saying what you feel.
- Confront annoyances in interpersonal relationships as they arise rather than allowing them to accumulate in intensity or building resentment.
- Take responsibility for your part in an interpersonal conflict.

Often, a combined approach using both antidepressant medications and psychotherapy is the most beneficial way to achieve effective and long-lasting relief from depression.

Psychotherapy is usually paid for by private insurers, Medicare, and Medicaid, but check with your policy to determine how mental health services are covered and what restrictions apply.

Other Treatment Options

In addition to antidepressant medications and psychotherapy, several other therapies may be appropriate for treating depression under certain circumstances.

ELECTROCONVULSIVE THERAPY

Sometimes, antidepressant medications, alone or in combination with psychotherapy, are not effective at relieving a person's depression. Fortunately, there is another option, a powerful treatment called electroconvulsive therapy, or ECT, also known as shock treatment. ECT was discovered by accident when people with both epilepsy and depression seemed to feel better after having a spontaneous seizure.

ECT uses a carefully controlled electrical current applied to two points on the patient's scalp. This current causes a temporary seizure that lasts for about a minute. Before treatment, the patient takes a muscle relaxant, and during the procedure, an anesthesiologist supervises the patient's breathing and heartbeat. The ECT treatments are repeated two or three times per week for a series of 6 to 20 treatments, on average, to achieve remission of the person's depressive symptoms. The exact mechanism by which ECT works is not known, but it likely restores the correct balance of electrochemical functions in the brain and thus relieves the depression.

ECT can cause short-term memory loss for events that occurred right before and after each treatment, but these memories usually return after a few hours. Medical screening for physical health must also be done prior to beginning ECT.

ECT has not been without controversy, as some people have complained of longer-lasting memory loss, even though careful research studies have not found any evidence of persistent memory loss six months after finishing a course of ECT.

Mental health professionals who regularly encounter severely depressed people tend to become believers in ECT's powerful effect after witnessing the recovery of not one but many people who had not responded to various other treatments. It is truly remarkable to see a person who previously could barely move or talk due to severe depression become restored to an active and conversational person after undergoing this type of treatment.

Private insurers, Medicare, and Medicaid all typically cover ECT for severe cases of depression.

ELECTRICAL STIMULATION THERAPIES

Another new and exciting way to treat depression involves various electrical stimulation therapies that deliver low-strength electrical stimulation to specific areas of the brain. In recent research trials, these methods have shown promise for treating selected individuals with severe, unremitting, or chronic depression.

Transcranial magnetic stimulation (TMS) involves holding a palm-sized device to the patient's scalp to deliver an oscillating magnetic field to a specific region of the brain. The oscillating magnetic field actually produces small electric currents on the brain surface. The patient receives 30 to 45 minutes of TMS daily for 20 to 30 sessions (or until the depression improves). This treatment does not require anesthesia and is performed in a psychiatrist's office, with the patient awake and alert. TMS does not cause muscle twitches as ECT does, but it can occasionally induce a seizure. It is also not as powerful at relieving depression as ECT.

TMS has had inconsistent results in relieving depression, which has limited its use to date. It is approved by the FDA for people who have not had relief from at least one adequate trial of an approved antidepressant medication, but it is not yet available in every community. Improvements in ways to consistently apply the stimulation to one specific brain area may improve its track record as a viable and readily available treatment in the future.

Vagus nerve stimulation (VNS) is another FDA-approved treatment for chronic unremitting depression. The technique is similar to one used for people with Parkinson disease to suppress the severe tremors that make eating soup with a spoon or signing one's name impossible. To provide relief from these debilitating tremors, tiny electrodes are implanted into specific areas of the spinal cord, and the wires are attached to a pacemaker-like device, also implanted under the skin and powered by a long-lasting battery. The device delivers an electrical signal to suppress the tremors.

In a person with depression, an electrode is surgically attached to the vagus nerve, which is a pencil-sized nerve bundle that leaves the brain at its base and carries nerve signals to the abdominal organs.

An implanted pacemaker causes the electrode to pulse a weak electrical signal upward through the vagus nerve and into the brain, where it appears to help stabilize the electrical activity of the brain, thus relieving depression. VNS is reserved for people who don't have relief from their depressive symptoms after at least four adequate trials of antidepressant drugs. A neurosurgeon must implant the device, and the patient must be monitored regularly so that the device can be adjusted for maximal benefit. VNS patients also need to remain on their antidepressant drugs. Many insurance companies are unwilling to pay for the procedure because, they argue, the evidence for its effectiveness is not strong enough, even though it is FDA approved. It is also costly (upwards of $20,000 at this writing). Nevertheless, for people with chronic, severe depression, VNS is an option worth considering.

Deep brain stimulation (DBS) is a procedure similar to VNS, but it involves implanting tiny electrodes deep within the brain at highly specific sites in both the right and left hemispheres. The connecting wires are attached to a pacemaker implanted under the skin of the upper chest. The theory behind this therapy is that a low-voltage pulsing current suppresses the activity in an area of the brain known as Broadman area 25. For some people, DBS has shown a remarkable antidepressant effect.

The VNS and DBS devices can be controlled by external electronic equipment that adjusts the voltage and other parameters to try to achieve the best results. Both VNS and DBS treatments require specialized aftercare as well as the initial surgery; they are thus quite expensive and only available at universities researching these procedures as well as larger medical centers. Electrical stimulation therapies are at the cutting edge of our understanding about how the brain works and how mood disorders can be successfully treated. The day may come when these techniques become more commonplace. For readers interested in further information, we have included some references in the resources at the end of the book.

PHOTOTHERAPY

A treatment for depression that uses bright white lights, called phototherapy, can relieve the symptoms of seasonal depression, or SAD. The artificial lights mimic the effect of sun exposure to receptors in the eyes and brain. Typically, someone with SAD sits, reads, or works with a light source of a specified brightness within 18 inches of his face for 15 to 60 minutes each day. To benefit from phototherapy for SAD, an individual needs to let the light bathe his face with his eyes open but doesn't need to look directly at the light source. Phototherapy light sources deliver a full-spectrum bright white light or blue light and have safety features to filter out ultraviolet light so that the individual is not sunburned or at increased risk of cataracts. People who use phototherapy for SAD usually don't need the therapy from May to October, but a few are exquisitely sensitive to seasonal changes in the sun's brightness and begin using SAD phototherapy in late August.

About 40 percent of individuals with severe SAD may need to take antidepressant medications or have psychotherapy as well as use phototherapy. Many people who have bipolar disorder or chronic major depression also experience a seasonal worsening of their mood that can often be improved by phototherapy.

HERBAL PREPARATIONS AND OTHER NATURAL SUBSTANCES

Several herbal preparations and other natural substances have been touted to have antidepressant effects. The preparations most commonly sold for their emotional or mental benefit are listed in table 1.5. Although there are anecdotal reports about benefits from people who consume these substances, anecdotes are not the same as rigorous scientific studies, so caution is warranted when considering herbal remedies.

Many of these preparations have not undergone rigorous scientific research with well-designed clinical trials to determine their antidepressant benefits. Also, herbal preparations are not considered to be drugs and therefore are not required to meet FDA standards for drug safety and efficacy. Without measurement standards, the concentration of active ingredients in these plant preparations can vary widely, so the potency of a particular herbal preparation may differ substantially among brands or even among batches made by the same company. The bottom line in considering the use of herbal preparations is the old adage "buyer beware."

In mild cases of anxiety or depression—and after taking into account the risk of side effects—herbal preparations may be safe to try,

Table 1.5. Some Popular Herbal Preparations with Purported Benefit for Depression and Anxiety

Name	Source	Purported benefit	Potential side effects
St. John's wort	*Hypericum*	Relieving depression, anxiety, or nausea	Nausea, heartburn, loose bowels, jitteriness, insomnia, fatigue
Kava	*Piper methisticum*	Relieving anxiety; giving a sense of conviviality and good-naturedness	Most commonly: gastrointestinal complaints, allergic skin reaction, headache, photosensitivity. Other complaints: restlessness, drowsiness, lack of energy, and tremors
Valerian root	*Valeriana officinalis* L.	Relieving anxiety or depression and providing relief for insomnia	Mild "hangover" effect at some doses

S̶ P. Brown and P. L. Gerbarg, "Herbs and Nutrients in the Treatment of D̶ , Anxiety, Insomnia, Migraine, and Obesity," *Journal of Psychiatric Prac-* t̶):75–91; *Consumer Health Digest*, "Omega-3 Fatty Acids and Depression" (2̶ w.consumerhealthdigest.com/omegafattyacids.htm.

b̶ ne advocates their use for serious or debilitating depression o̶ ty. They should never replace prescription medications for s̶ epression nor be combined with prescription drugs, because o̶ ble negative interactions and side effects.

u̶ are considering using an herbal preparation, speak with y̶ ctor first to be sure it is safe for you and won't have adverse i̶ ions with other medications you may be taking.

 other natural substance, omega-3 fatty acid, deserves a brief r̶ n. The omega-3 fatty acid story is an interesting one: the American diet has seen a drastic decline in these fatty acids, which are derived mostly from fish oil and certain seed oils like flaxseed oil. One-fifth of the dry weight of human brain tissue is made up of omega-3 fatty acids, so consuming enough omega-3 in the diet may have something to do with maintaining good brain function, including mood. Omega-3 fatty acids seem to help stabilize cell membrane functions in brain cells and may have other effects, such as blocking inflammation, which can worsen mood. In fact, in cultures that eat more fish, like the Japanese culture, the rates of depression are statistically lower. Various manufacturers produce omega-3 supplements as an oil in soft gel caps, and some use a steam process to remove the fishy odor. Note, however, that omega-3 supplements are not intended to be a treatment for depression by themselves, but are an adjunct to more traditional treatments provided by a qualified professional.

Long-Term Management

Depression is an illness that tends to recur, and the more episodes you have in your lifetime, the greater your chances of having another one. Research has shown that people who have had three or more episodes can disrupt this pattern by staying on antidepressant medication lifelong. If continued medication doesn't prevent future episodes, it will at least decrease their severity.

Maintenance psychotherapy can also help prevent new episodes of depression, particularly in individuals whose depression stems from difficulties with maintaining mutually satisfying relationships, such as people who struggle with chronic marital discord. Regular "booster" sessions of psychotherapy, such as once a month, can help remind individuals to keep practicing the new methods they have learned for handling problems rather than revert back to the old ones that contributed to being depressed.

For a small minority of people with depression, ECT is the only treatment that seems to provide relief, and receiving maintenance ECT once a month for a lifetime is a legitimate option that can keep the depression from returning.

Lessening the Chances of Becoming Depressed

Problems and stresses are inevitable in life. Everyone copes differently with problems, and how well you are able to cope can have a profound impact on whether you feel demoralized, helpless, and depressed or optimistic and determined to work through problems and seek life's satisfactions. People who can focus on the latter more often help reduce their stress and therefore lessen the risk of developing serious depression. By knowing what you can do, you can take a more proactive approach to keeping minor depression from turning into more serious or incapacitating depression.

Maintaining a healthy lifestyle clearly helps reduce the stresses that trigger depression. Commonsense lifestyle strategies include

- eating a nutritionally balanced diet
- getting adequate sleep
- maintaining a healthy weight
- minimizing the amount of alcohol you drink or recreational drugs you consume
- pursuing satisfying social relationships and social outlets
- getting aerobic exercise
- keeping a balance between work and leisure that allows time for emotionally restorative and pleasurable activities

An adequate social support system is a definite factor in lessening the chances of developing depression. For example, married people are at less risk for depression than nonmarried people, and lonely or isolated individuals are at higher risk.

There are many activities that older people can consider pursuing to help them change aspects of their lifestyle or broaden their social network. Finding and pursuing activities that interest you can be particularly important after you retire from the workforce and no longer have regular interaction with colleagues, customers, clients, or the public. Many activities are available at community centers, seniors' centers, and other venues. Here are some ideas to consider:

- Learn and practice a mindfulness activity, such as yoga, meditation, or tai chi.
- Find a hobby or join a group, such as a book club, related to your interests.
- Participate in religious or spiritual activities.
- Join a gym or take an exercise class.
- Keep a journal or diary.
- Pursue artistic activities, such as taking classes or attending performances.
- Volunteer in your community.
- Get a pet.

- Travel to a place you've always wanted to visit.
- See a therapist or counselor to explore problem-solving strategies and seek new ways to cope with problems you're encountering.

People who are developing memory loss may be less able to solve day-to-day problems and identify ways to improve their lifestyle, and they are more likely to feel stuck or hopeless at times. These individuals may need more help from others to solve problems or more encouragement to structure their routines so that they avoid feeling demoralized. We discuss issues with memory loss in relation to depression and anxiety in chapter 3.

■ ■ ■

If You Are Concerned That You May Be Depressed

- Don't ignore or dismiss your feelings.
- Tell a family member or friend.
- Speak to a member of the clergy or someone else you respect in your community.
- Visit your primary care doctor or mental health care provider.
- Go to a nearby hospital or emergency room in severe cases or if you have suicidal thoughts.
- If you feel like you can't cope any longer, call a crisis line or suicide prevention line. The phone numbers of some national organizations are listed in the resources section of this book.

Suggestions for Family Members and Caregivers

If you are concerned about depression in another person, or if someone confides in you about symptoms that may signal depression, you can do several things to help:

- Learn to recognize the signs and symptoms of depression in older people.
- Listen carefully to someone telling you about symptoms.
- Suggest that the person see a doctor. Offer to make the appointment and go with the person to the appointment.

- Learn more about depression from this book and the resources listed at the end of the book.
- Spend time with the person and be supportive. Offer encouragement and hope.
- Invite the person out for social activities.
- Offer to help with chores like grocery shopping, cleaning, or home maintenance.
- Take care of yourself if you are the caregiver of a person with depression. Caregivers and other people who live with a person with depression are at risk of developing depression themselves because of the stress of being around someone who is irritable, uncooperative, and critical, as many depressed people can be.
- If someone you're concerned about refuses help for what appears to be depression, you can explain the situation to his doctor. Although the current privacy laws forbid doctors from talking to other people about their patients, you can convey your concerns and leave it up to the doctor to use the information to explore further at the person's next appointment. For example, you can write a letter or call the doctor's office and state who you are, why you are making contact, and that you realize you won't get any response or discussion in return.
- In critical situations, when a person not only appears to be depressed but also is in apparent danger of hurting himself or others, you can call your local police or emergency room and ask about your state's procedure for initiating an involuntary commitment for mental health evaluation and treatment. Each state has its own laws, but they all share the basic concept of providing involuntary care for someone who refuses care due to mental illness and who is at high risk of injury, illness, or death if protected care (usually in a psychiatric unit) is not provided.

TWO

What You Need to Know about Anxiety

All humans are hardwired to experience anxiety, for good reason. When confronted by a menacing dog with teeth bared, our nervous system automatically prepares us for "fight or flight." This automatic response happens because special glands release the hormone epinephrine (also called adrenaline) into the bloodstream. Epinephrine increases heart rate and raises blood pressure. It also restricts blood flow to the gut—digestion can wait for later—and shunts blood to our muscles, making them ready for action. Epinephrine prepares our brain to take quick and decisive action. We feel "on edge" because our sharpened senses are ready to allow us either to fight in self-protection or to escape. The accompanying emotional reaction, which has evolved over millennia to preserve the lives of mammals, is anxiety.

Although anxiety is normal, excessive anxiety is not and can be just as bothersome and debilitating as depression. Triggers that can lead to anxiety include medical illness, mental distress, perceived threats to health or safety, and various substances, including caffeine and some medications. Sometimes anxiety occurs with no obvious trigger, and it can vary in intensity. People who experience chronically high levels of anxiety that interfere with their ability to function socially or at work are said to have an anxiety disorder.

Only in the past 15 years have researchers begun to focus specifically on how anxiety manifests in older people and what triggers may be unique to older age. Certainly, individuals who are vulnerable to an anxiety disorder in their 20s and 30s tend to remain vulnerable to anxiety throughout their lives and may require lifelong treatment. Often, however, anxiety flares up in some older people who haven't previously experienced excessive anxiety or an anxiety disorder, and the trigger is frequently a serious medical problem or disability, such as a heart attack or loss of vision.

In this chapter, we discuss the link between anxiety and depression, how to recognize anxiety issues and disorders in older adults, the triggers that can cause anxiety, and the range of treatment and management options, which include medication, psychotherapy, avoidance of anxiety-inducing substances, and lifestyle changes to reduce stress.

The Link between Anxiety and Depression

Many people experience anxiety and depression at the same time, and although some of the symptoms overlap, these illnesses are distinct. Anxiety and depression can each lead to the other developing. For example, somebody who feels nervous or anxious all the time can become depressed if she feels restricted in her home or work life by her anxiety symptoms. The physical symptoms of anxiety, such as a racing heart, tense muscles, lack of sleep, and poor concentration, can all leave a person feeling less capable than usual and, if they persist, can contribute to developing depression. Conversely, somebody who has depression may develop anxieties about her inability to work or function in her home life.

When severe anxiety and depression coexist, people experience a very uncomfortable state of mind. In these cases, often described as agitated depression, individuals pace, wring their hands, and are unable to get comfortable. They feel helpless and hopeless about finding relief. Agitated depression increases the risk of suicide.

When someone has both depression and anxiety, regardless of which one came first, the treatment of one may ease the other. For example, the serotonin-boosting medications used for depression also have antianxiety properties, although they can take a week or more to start lowering anxiety. In many instances, separate treatments may be used, with antidepressant medication and ideally psychotherapy to treat the depression and simultaneous use of antianxiety medication (typically benzodiazepines, discussed later in this chapter) to quickly control the anxiety. Eventually, the benzodiazepines can be stopped, once the seratonin-boosting antidepressants achieve their full effect, which can take one to four weeks.

Recognizing Excessive Anxiety and Anxiety Disorders

Since childhood, Phillip had had symptoms of anxiety. Going to school had been a difficult adjustment for him, as he was shy and anxious around other children. As an older child, he fretted over tests and having to stand up and read assignments aloud. He never received a diagnosis or treatment, though, and learned to compensate by immersing himself in his studies. He graduated from university as an engineer and got a job in a large company. Phillip had a reputation as a hard worker and an innovative problem solver, and he met with a lot of success in his chosen field. When he was anxious about a problem in one of his engineering projects, he would stay up late working on it until he solved it. At age 65, Phillip retired and spent much of his time making fine furniture in his basement woodworking shop.

Phillip had been diagnosed with prostate cancer at age 62 and had elected to have it treated with surgery and radiation. The checkup appointments indicated that the treatment had been successful; however, five years later, at age 67, Phillip experienced lower back pain, and an x-ray showed what was likely metastasized (spreading) prostate cancer. His doctor explained the various treatment options, and Phillip also explored options on the Internet. Despite spending hours researching, he couldn't seem to find much to feel reassured about. The more he read, the more anxious he became. In the days after the new diagnosis, Phillip sometimes felt like he couldn't get his breath and thought he might be having a heart attack. Other times he felt he just had to get outside for more air.

Phillip was experiencing panic attacks brought on by his worries related to the spread of his cancer. Phillip's lifelong anxiety, though undiagnosed until this point in his life, was determined to be generalized anxiety disorder. His anxious tendency made him especially vulnerable to the brief periods of intense and frightening anxiety called panic attacks. Fortunately, Phillip returned to his primary care doctor and received treatment for his anxieties as well as his cancer.

People often experience anxiety as a combination of mental symptoms (such as fearfulness, apprehension, wariness, irritability, poor concentration, and being easily startled) and physical symptoms (such as muscle tension, rapid heart rate, rapid breathing, sweating, feeling weak or light-headed, and sometimes diarrhea). As we've said, when these symptoms occur in response to actual danger, they are normal, but experienced frequently or for long periods when little or no danger exists, they are classified as excessive anxiety. If the symptoms interfere with a person's ability to function at daily tasks or at work, she may have an anxiety disorder, the most common being generalized anxiety disorder.

Generalized Anxiety Disorder

Generalized anxiety disorder, or GAD, is the condition experienced by people who are chronically overanxious about a situation or whose anxiety is triggered by little or no provocation to the point that their symptoms interfere with their jobs or social lives. People with GAD are persistently and unrealistically worried, often about minor or everyday problems, and they frequently expect disaster. GAD is the most prevalent anxiety disorder, with 2 to 7 percent of older adults suffering from it at any one time. The condition often stems from worries about money, work, family, health, and, particularly in the frail elderly, a fear of falling. GAD is diagnosed if the persistent worry occurs on most days over a six-month period.

About 60 percent of people diagnosed with GAD have major depression (as described in chapter 1), which brought on the anxiety. The state of depression amounts to a stress in which the anxiety develops. For example, imagine someone who is severely depressed and can't go to work for many weeks. She could easily become highly anxious when her sick leave time begins to run out, and she realizes that she could lose her job if she can't return to work. In individuals with co-occurring GAD and depression, resolving the depression usually also resolves the anxiety symptoms.

Panic Attacks

A panic attack involves a heightened sense of anxiety that is so intense, people experiencing it often believe they are losing their mind, having a heart attack, or facing imminent death. Panic attacks often send people to the emergency room, where a heart attack is ruled out and they receive a medication such as lorazepam (brand name Ativan) to calm them. Most panic attacks follow a period of intense emotional stress. Depression is one stress that can bring on panic attacks.

Panic Disorder

Some people experience recurring panic attacks with no obvious provocation or stressful situation. Their nervous system appears to initiate the "fight or flight" response without a trigger. A person who has spontaneous panic attacks without warning is diagnosed with panic disorder.

Having a panic attack can be so frightening that a person will do almost anything to avoid having another. As a result, people often avoid the place (or places) where their panic attacks have occurred. Panic disorder is the most common cause of agoraphobia, which comes from the Greek words *agora*, meaning "open spaces," and *phobia*, meaning "fear." As people who experience panic attacks progressively avoid more and more places where their attacks have occurred, they eventually become fearful of leaving their home altogether. In some severe cases, individuals have been trapped in their homes for 10 years or more and have depended on family members to survive.

Phobias

Phobias are anxiety syndromes that involve an intense fear of places, animals, or situations. The fear is typically strong and often irrational (to an outside observer). People with phobias try to avoid the object or situation that they fear, and if they can't, they experience anxiety symptoms like panic, rapid heart rate, shortness of breath, trembling, tense muscles, and a strong desire to escape the situation.

Phobias are generally classified into three groups:

- Agoraphobia, the fear of being outside or of particular places
- Social phobia, the fear of being misjudged, accused, or embarrassed in social situations or of meeting new people
- Specific phobias, the fear of particular things or situations, such as spiders (arachnophobia), flying (aerophobia), confined spaces (claustrophobia), height (acrophobia), or cancer (carcinophobia)

Phobias are relatively common, with about 8 percent of adults in the United States experiencing one sometime during their lives.

The incidence of phobias increases slightly from ages 18 to 65, and women have phobias from two to four times more frequently than men.

Post-traumatic Stress Disorder

Post-traumatic stress disorder (PTSD) occurs in individuals who have endured a highly frightening or life-threatening situation, such as witnessing the carnage from a disaster, combat situation, accident, or other terrifying event. People with PTSD can feel like they are reliving the event and can experience intense emotions and physical symptoms, as well as the desire to avoid anything that reminds them of the traumatic situation. Even when successfully treated, PTSD can recur later in an individual's life if a similar experience or reminder of the original trauma occurs.

Obsessive-Compulsive Disorder

Obsessive-compulsive disorder (OCD) typically occurs in one of two ways. Individuals with OCD often have thoughts that repeat in their mind like an uncontrollable broken record. Alternatively, people with OCD can have ritualistic or compulsive behaviors, such as counting, ordering, checking, or cleaning items in their surroundings. Examples of compulsive behaviors are repeatedly washing hands, checking that the stove is turned off, or checking that doors are locked. Some individuals with OCD have predominantly obsessive thinking or predominantly compulsive behaviors, while others display both signs of the disorder. People with OCD frequently order their belongings by size or color or turn everyday tasks, such as bathing, into compulsory rituals. These rituals involve self-imposed sequences of events that must take place in strict order to prevent intolerable anxiety. In severe cases, people with these rituals can require three hours or more just to take a bath or shower.

OCD is considered an anxiety disorder because anxiety levels rise unless the person suffering from this affliction carries out the compulsive behaviors that temporarily reduce the anxiety. For example, people with a compulsive need to check the door to make sure it's locked will sit down after checking the door and know in their mind that they just checked it, yet a small part of their brain tells them that doubt still remains. Their anxiety levels begin to rise as they ponder whether the door really is locked, despite having checked it a few minutes earlier, until they feel compelled to check the door once more. Doing so temporarily relieves the anxiety, but then the cycle begins again.

Obsessive-compulsive disorders differ from obsessive-compulsive personality disorder, or OCPD, which is characterized by life-long traits of fastidiousness, inordinate attention to detail, and inflexible thinking, such that most life decisions are considered to be black and white rather than shades of gray. People with OCPD are usually not as impaired as those with OCD and don't display the repetitive checking behaviors or rituals.

As OCD tends to be a lifelong disorder that usually begins in childhood or early adulthood, older individuals who show features of OCD have usually had them for many years. The symptoms can interact with the aging process, however, and affect an individual's ability to cope with the disorder, as happened in the case of Stanley.

Stanley was not diagnosed with OCD until he was in the eighth grade, but looking back, he had been showing signs of the disorder much earlier. He recalled spending hours alone in his room organizing his toys by color, size, and shape. He'd had rigid daily routines and food preferences and dislikes. In junior high, he needed two hours to prepare for school every morning, going through unbreakable rituals of showering and grooming. Eventually, the school counselor encouraged Stanley to see a psychiatrist, and, with his parents' consent, he was started on medication that made him less rigid in his routines.

Stanley finished high school, attended a two-year college program, and landed a job as an accountant in a large business. The managers liked his steady work ethic and attention to details, and he worked at the same business until he retired. In his 30s, he married a woman his mother introduced him to, and they had two children.

Even though he continued to take medication, Stanley's OCD symptoms interfered with his life in certain ways. He would get obsessed with collecting things, often expensive items like rare stamps, which brought him into conflict with his wife. She also complained that he was so rigid in his political and religious beliefs that he could never see other people's points of view and was increasingly difficult to live with.

After 25 years of marriage, and as their second child graduated from high school, his wife asked for a divorce, stating that she couldn't stand living with him any longer.

After retiring several years later, Stanley lived by himself in an apartment and took up collecting electric trains. He amassed a robust collection that began to feel out of control, even for him. He had trains in unopened boxes that he had ordered and traded online. His children visited him dutifully but also found him hard to relate to, given his rigid views, and both children felt they could never manage having him live with them.

Then Stanley had a heart attack, which led to depression, and his rigid thinking seemed to get worse. He had a hard time making even small decisions, and he got behind on paying bills, although he kept buying electric trains when he came across a rare one. As his finances spun out of control, his children felt obligated to step in and try to sort it out. They confronted him with the obvious conclusion that he needed to sell his trains to pay off his debts. Stanley couldn't bring himself to sell them, but he allowed his son to do so. He eventually agreed to move into a personal care home, where he could get assistance with medications, have meals provided for him, and, most important, have limits on his collecting habits.

Risk Factors for Developing Excessive Anxiety or an Anxiety Disorder

As with depression, some people are more vulnerable than others to anxiety. Studies have shown that heredity, or genetic makeup, can increase a person's susceptibility to developing an anxiety disorder. Life experiences can also set people up for experiencing excessive anxiety in certain situations. For example, enduring a traumatic event, such as being bitten by a dog, can predispose a vulnerable individual to greater anxiety, in this case being anxious around all dogs. Anxiety can also result from the stress of experiencing a personal dilemma, being involved in a dispute in an important relationship, facing a threatened or actual loss, or experiencing a personal injury or illness.

Some people also argue that modern society has spawned additional reasons for anxiety—overcrowding, traffic, rigid work schedules, productivity requirements, sensory bombardment, sleep deprivation, overconsumption of coffee and energy drinks, and the generally increasing complexity of our modern world. The stresses induced by these phenomena have caused many individuals to feel increasingly anxious under various circumstances.

Too Much Caffeine

Many people enjoy drinking tea, coffee, or other caffeinated beverages; however, overconsumption of caffeine—which is the most commonly consumed stimulant—frequently leads to excessive anxiety. The caffeine sources we're most familiar with are caffeinated beverages, but caffeine is also in products like chocolate, some candies, ice creams, and medications, as shown in table 2.1.

The concentration of caffeine varies enormously, especially in coffee and tea, because different brands, brewing times, and pro-

Table 2.1. The Caffeine Content in Common Foods and Beverages

Item	Size	Caffeine content, milligrams
Coffee	8 ounce cup	
brewed		95–200
instant		25–175
espresso		400–600
decaffeinated		2–12
Tea	8 ounce cup	
black		30–120
green		20–30
Hot chocolate	8 ounce cup	2–8
Iced tea	12 ounce can	5–30
Cola soft drink	12 ounce can	35–70
Energy drink	8 ounce can	80–100
Chocolate	40 gram bar	10–30
Coffee ice cream	8 ounce scoop	40–60
Medications (e.g., pain relievers, cold medicines)	1 tablet	30–200

Sources: Mayo Foundation for Medical Education and Research, Caffeine Content for Coffee, Tea, Soda and More (2009), www.mayoclinic.com/health/caffeine/AN01211; and Food and Drug Administration, *Caffeine in My Home: Caffeine and Your Body* (2007), publication UCM205286.pdf at www.fda.gov.

cessing methods all contribute to the caffeine content. On average, a cup of coffee has 100 to 200 milligrams of caffeine. Some people have reported drinking as many as 20 cups of coffee daily, which puts their caffeine consumption as high as 4,000 milligrams in a single day, without including other foods or drinks they might be consuming. Although 20 cups of coffee a day is probably excessive by most people's standards, it can still be surprisingly easy to take in more than the recommended daily maximum of 500–600 milligrams of caffeine. If you know that you suffer from excessive anxiety, or if you have unexplained headaches, have difficulty sleeping, or feel edgy, it may be helpful to carefully tally your daily intake of caffeine and other stimulants and then decide where to cut back.

Medical Conditions

Several medical conditions can cause anxiety or increase the intensity of anxiety symptoms in older individuals:

- Heart problems, including chest pain (angina), irregular heartbeat (arrhythmia), decreased ability to pump or circulate enough blood (congestive heart failure), faulty heart valve (valvular disease), and heart attack; heart attacks in particular can make people worry about having another, possibly fatal, heart attack, as well as making them hyper-attentive to every chest sensation they feel
- Lung problems, including emphysema (chronic obstructive pulmonary disease, or COPD), asthma, and hyperventilation syndrome (when someone breathes very quickly and deeply and becomes dizzy as a result); these conditions can give people the sense of not being able to catch their breath
- Hormonal problems, including diabetes, high blood sugar (hyperglycemia), low blood sugar (hypoglycemia), overactive thyroid gland (hyperthyroidism), underactive thyroid gland (hypothyroidism), and excess adrenaline (called pheochromocytoma, a tumor of the gland that produces adrenaline)
- Neurological problems, including dizziness (vertigo) and seizure disorders
- Gut problems, primarily peptic ulcers (erosions in the lining of the stomach or small intestine)

- Urinary incontinence, which can make an person fearful of going out and having an accident or not being near a restroom
- Vision loss, which increases anxiety about getting lost, being unable to recognize people or hazards, and being unable to drive
- Any condition that makes walking more difficult or increases the fear of falling, including arthritis, stroke, diminished feeling in the feet, and loss of vision; having to go out on snowy or icy surfaces also causes anxiety, and people who use a cane, walker, wheelchair, or scooter often become anxious about transporting the equipment and negotiating curbs and doorways
- Any illness or physical disability that limits function, driving, walking, perceived independence, or the ability to pursue social interactions

Prescribed and Over-the-Counter Medications

Some people experience anxiety symptoms when taking certain prescription or over-the-counter medications, shown in table 2.2. Sometimes the combination of an over-the-counter cold preparation and another medication can cause excessive anxiety, panic attacks, or even paranoid psychosis (hallucinations or delusions). If you develop anxi-

Table 2.2. Medications That May Cause Anxiety Symptoms

Type of medication	Examples
Prescription	
Asthma	Albuterol, salmeterol, and theophylline
Blood pressure	Methyldopa
Stimulants	Dexedrine (amphetamine) and Ritalin (methylphenidate)
Steroids	Cortisone, dexamethasone, and prednisone
Thyroid	Levothyroxine
Others	Phenytoin, levodopa, quinidine, some antidepressants
Over-the-counter	
Containing caffeine	Anacin, Empirin, Excedrin, No-Doz, and cough medicines
Decongestants	Phenylephrine (e.g., Sudafed PE)

Source: Healthwise, Medicines That Can Cause Anxiety (2008), www.revolution health.com/conditions/mental-behavioral-health/anxiety/causes/medications-cause -anxiety.

ety symptoms, especially after taking a new medication, discuss the symptoms with your doctor immediately.

Complications of Anxiety

As well as complications like social isolation and avoidance of places or situations to the point that it interferes with an individual's life, people with chronic anxiety are at increased risk of developing chronic medical problems. Medical problems that can be caused by a prolonged high anxiety include high blood pressure (hypertension), ulcers, inflammation of the colon (colitis), and migraine headaches, as well as depression. Some people attempt to relieve their chronic anxiety by drinking more alcohol or taking (and often becoming addicted to) prescription medications, both of which add another complication to the treatment of anxiety and other medical problems.

Getting Treatment for Anxiety Symptoms and Disorders

Various treatment and management options are available to help people who experience anxiety symptoms or an anxiety disorder. Medications are typically prescribed for individuals who are diagnosed with generalized anxiety disorder, obsessive-compulsive disorder, or panic disorder, as well as for people with excessive anxiety that isn't diagnosed as a specific disorder. Counseling, or psychotherapy, can help people develop strategies to cope with situations or issues that induce their anxiety, such as grief, a strained marriage, or a difficult boss. A combination of medications and psychotherapy can often be the most effective.

Medications

Numerous medications, shown in table 2.3, are effective for treating anxiety disorders, with SSRIs and benzodiazepines being the most commonly used medications in older adults. Generalized anxiety disorder and panic disorder can usually be treated effectively with serotonin-boosting medications (SSRIs or SNRIs) administered for two to four weeks for a full effect. These medications are often successful at reducing the intensity of anxiety symptoms, a bit like turning down the volume of a stereo. These same medications have also been approved by the FDA for treating obsessive-compulsive disorder, but

Table 2.3. Common Medications for Anxiety Disorders and
Possible Side Effects

Drug category	Examples (brand name in parentheses)	Possible side effects
Selective serotonin reuptake inhibitors (SSRIs)	citalopram (Celexa), paroxetine (Paxil), fluoxetine (Prozac)	Nausea, headache, sweating, sexual problems
Benzodiazepines	lorazepam (Ativan), alprazolam (Xanax)	Sedation, unsteady gait, falling, confusion, physiological dependence
Serotonin and norepinephrine reuptake inhibitors (SNRIs)	venlafaxine XR (Effexor XR), desvenlafaxine (Pristiq), duloxetine (Cymbalta)	Nausea, headache, sweating, sexual problems, high blood pressure
Mild tranquilizers	buspirone (Buspar)	Light-headedness, balance problems, incoordination

they generally require higher doses and at least three months before
determining if they will be effective.

Benzodiazepine medications are potent drugs that act quickly to
relieve anxiety, and they are safe and effective when administered
properly. They are not preferred for long-term treatment, however,
because they can have several negative side effects, particularly in older
individuals. These side effects include oversedation, an increased risk
of falling due to impaired balance or unsteady gait, memory disturbance, and confusion. The benzodiazepine medications are so effective that many individuals become psychologically dependent on
them. The nervous system can become physiologically dependent
on them as well, resulting in severe withdrawal symptoms if they are
discontinued too abruptly. Withdrawal symptoms can include sweating, nervousness, rapid heartbeat, high blood pressure, irritability,
and in the worst cases, seizures and even death. For these reasons,
chronic use of this class of medications is discouraged in favor of
short-term use with a gradual tapering to zero. Sometimes avoiding
long-term use of benzodiazepines is not possible, however, as some
individuals can't tolerate the side effects of alternative medications
such as the SSRIs.

Psychotherapy

Psychotherapy, which we described at length in chapter 1, can help people with anxiety explore coping strategies, as well as reveal hidden or masked stresses that are causing or contributing to anxiety.

> Julie was in her mid-60s when she began to experience regular panic attacks while crossing a bridge that led out of the town where she lived. Frightened by her racing heart, she went to her doctor, who suggested she see a psychotherapist. Through a process of exploratory psychotherapy, her therapist helped reveal her mixed feelings and thoughts about whether to stay with or leave her husband. Julie was unaware of her mental association between crossing the bridge out of town and her thoughts about leaving her marriage. This association triggered her panic attacks while crossing the bridge. In other words, crossing the bridge held a personalized, symbolic meaning for Julie. By exploring her ambivalence toward her marriage, the connection to crossing the bridge became clear in her mind, and her tendency to panic on the bridge subsided. She consciously decided to face her marital issues and encourage her husband to join her in marital counseling.

One type of psychotherapy, called cognitive behavioral therapy (CBT), can teach individuals with OCD how to better control their thinking, rather than letting their repetitive thoughts or compulsive behaviors control them. This treatment takes time and practice to learn and become proficient at the techniques, but when it's successful, the symptoms can be as effectively relieved as with the use of medication. Sometimes, people manage to control their symptoms using only the learned techniques without needing any medication.

CBT can also help patients who have developed the habit of avoiding various places for fear of having a panic attack. A CBT therapist will guide and encourage such individuals to increase the distance they travel outside their comfort zone in ever widening circles. The therapist helps them confront their fears of having another panic attack in a given situation and provides tools for them to learn to endure the initial anxiety associated with exploring outside their comfort zone. The goal is to continue to widen the variety of social settings they can endure without having a new panic attack, and with time and practice, these individuals regain confidence, allowing them to travel farther away from home without having any more panic attacks.

This technique can be used for individuals who have developed a phobia as well. Phobias can result from dramatic events that trigger a state of intense fear. For example, imagine someone who encounters a snake in the woods and is terrified of being bitten. This traumatic event could lead to a snake phobia in a vulnerable person, who then avoids all wooded or grassy areas where snakes might live. A therapist might go through a process of systematic desensitization by having the person look at photographs of snakes in books, discuss their habitat, and learn the differences between harmless and poisonous species. As the phobic person becomes more comfortable with the subject of snakes in general, she would be encouraged to gradually increase her exposure to them. She may take a trip to the zoo to view a snake behind glass and then possibly handle a live, nonpoisonous snake under the guidance of a trained handler as a final step. These techniques can diffuse the intensity of a phobic anxiety and, in the best outcomes, can actually cure the phobia.

Herbal Preparations

Over-the-counter herbal preparations, including valerian root and kava, have been described as having calming properties. We discussed these compounds, and particularly some cautions about their use, in chapter 1, and we refer you to that section if you are considering using a herbal preparation.

Lessening the Chances of Developing an Anxiety Disorder

For individuals with anxiety, making several lifestyle changes can help relieve their symptoms. In fact, all of us who lead stressful lives in modern society could benefit from regularly practicing or using one or more of the following techniques:

- Get regular physical exercise to increase your fitness and help you deal more effectively with stress.
- Use relaxation techniques to benefit both physical and mental health. Numerous techniques can be practiced at home or in a class, such as guided imagery, transcendental meditation, tai chi, and yoga.

- Avoid or cut back your intake of alcohol and caffeine; both can make anxiety worse.
- Quit smoking. Although the effects of nicotine are complex (sometimes calming and sometimes stimulating), nicotine definitely has immediate effects on the brain and nervous system, which reinforces continued use to get the sought-after effect (addiction).
- Get enough quality sleep so that you are well rested and able to deal more effectively with life's daily challenges with less anxiety-provoking distress.
- Manage your time effectively to avoid the stress that comes from being overscheduled and having too many things to do in too little time.
- Develop and use good organizational skills to control the stress of misplacing important items and documents or procrastinating until deadlines loom and anxiety increases.
- Maintain a strong social support network to connect with others and share experiences. Social interaction and relationships are important to mental health. Supportive friends who are good listeners can buffer the intensity of stressful situations.

■ ■ ■

If You Are Concerned That You May Have an Anxiety Disorder

- Start by speaking to a family member, friend, or religious leader about your concerns. Merely verbalizing to another concerned person can help.
- Write down your feelings of anxiety to try to analyze when they occur and if there seems to be a trigger, and pay attention to what, if anything, eases the feelings of anxiety.
- Make an appointment to see your primary care doctor or other health care provider.
- Join an anxiety support group. See the resources listed at the end of this book.
- Consider working with a mental health provider to learn better coping strategies.

Suggestions for Family Members and Caregivers

If you are concerned about anxiety in another person, or if someone tells you about her anxiety symptoms, you can help in several ways.

- Learn to recognize the signs and symptoms of anxiety in older people.
- Listen carefully to someone telling you about symptoms.
- Ask specific questions, such as:
  Are you aware of what triggers your anxious feelings?
  Is something in your life causing you concern?
  Do you find it difficult to put things out of your mind?
- Suggest that the person see a doctor, and offer to go along to the appointment.
- Learn more about anxiety issues and disorders from this book and from the resources listed at the end of this book.
- Help out with daily activities that may be increasing the person's stress level.
- Invite the person on social outings.

Part II

Handling Challenges
over the Next Thirty Years

THREE

Coping with Memory Loss

As people age, they frequently worry about their memory. If they forget someone's name or misplace their keys, many people automatically worry that they are losing their memory, and especially that they may be in the beginning stages of Alzheimer disease. Age-related memory loss, however, or memory glitches—like not being able to recall a word—are entirely normal, provided that they don't interfere with day-to-day life. Typically, people know that they're a little more absent minded than they used to be, and they can even joke about it. On the other hand, people with memory loss for a reason other than aging may realize that something has changed but can't figure out what it is. They may also try to hide or gloss over their memory slips. Eventually, their memory loss can make it difficult for them to function in their daily lives.

In this chapter, we discuss the possible causes of memory loss and other impairments to brain function, focusing on Alzheimer disease and other dementias as well as the available treatments and management strategies. Many types of dementia can lead to depression, because as the disease progresses, mood structures and circuits become damaged within the brain. For example, a serious bout of depression can be the first indicator of the onset of Alzheimer disease. However, dementia and depression don't always coexist, and with similar symptoms, it can be difficult to distinguish them, so we compare the features of both diseases. Because of the severe impairment that can occur with dementia, we also describe strategies for caregivers. Last, we provide tips for proactively protecting your brain and memory.

What Is Normal Memory Loss and What Isn't?

The brain stores information in different ways. The most familiar categories of memory are short-term and long-term memory. Short-term memory involves being able to recall a phone number long enough to write it down, while long-term memory involves permanently fixing information so that the person can recall it weeks, years, or even decades later. Memories that are repeated, or "overlearned," such as multiplication tables and commonly used phone numbers, become more permanent than less used memories. Adequate sleep seems to be an important factor in transferring short-term memories to long-term. If particular memories are not used, they will decay over time.

Normal declines in memory begin at around age 30. As people age, there is a small but measurable drop-off in various memory capacities and in their ability to learn new material. Aging can also make it harder for people to recall pieces of information stored in their memory. Short-term memories tend to be affected by age more than long-term memories. For example, you may forget the name of someone you met earlier in the day, but you can easily recall your childhood best friend's name. These mild memory changes are entirely normal.

Normal memory loss doesn't usually change much over time, whereas memory loss associated with dementia tends to get progressively worse, often over the short time span of several months. Memory loss sufficient to merit a diagnosis of dementia is never normal, no matter the person's age.

People with Alzheimer disease and sometimes other dementias experience memory loss, but it can also result from other medical conditions unrelated to aging, including mental illnesses, like depression and anxiety, or minor head injury. Memory loss is a side effect of some medications and can also result from chronic alcoholism and even poor nutrition. In some of these instances, the loss can be stopped or reversed. For example, as discussed in the first two chapters of this book, both depression and anxiety can be effectively treated, so if memory loss occurs as a symptom of depression, relieving the depression will likely alleviate the memory loss. If medication side effects are to blame for memory problems, then different drugs can be tried.

Recognizing Dementia

Frank retired from his job at a manufacturing facility, where he had been employed for 35 years. He had worked hard and provided well for his family on his modest income, even managing to send his three children to college. All three were married, and Frank and his wife, Lois, had five grandchildren. Frank had a gentle disposition and was fond of animals, much to his grandkids' delight, as they all had pets.

After a few years of retirement, Lois noticed that Frank was becoming more irritable and argumentative with her. He argued over her spending habits, even though she was taking the same frugal approach she always had. What really upset Lois was his accusation that she was having an affair. Once, Frank had been so angry with Lois that he had locked her out of the house for an hour on a cold fall day. Later, he acted like nothing had happened and seemed back to his old self.

When their daughter Wendy tearfully confided to them that she had decided to seek a divorce, Lois tried to be consoling and supportive, but after Wendy left, Frank became angry with Lois and berated her once again, saying that they would now need to support Wendy, and it would drain their life savings, landing them in the "poor house." Lois tried explaining that Wendy had not asked for any financial help and that her current husband had a good job and would likely be paying child support if he and Wendy did divorce. Frank persisted in his view, unconvinced by her logical arguments.

Lois was embarrassed to tell her children about Frank's change in personality and behavior, because she didn't want to diminish their view of their father. She did speak with a geriatric psychiatrist, though, who encouraged Lois to have Frank see a doctor. Indeed, Frank was suffering from Alzheimer disease. His personality change and aggressive behavior were signs of executive dysfunction, a problem with one area of cognitive ability affected by Alzheimer disease. (We describe executive dysfunction later in this chapter.)

Frank began taking medication, which calmed him. He continued to enjoy playing with his grandkids and their pets. Meanwhile, his family learned about the illness and what to expect. They also stopped having complex, upsetting conversations in Frank's presence because he couldn't grasp their intended meaning.

Dementia is a general term used to describe deterioration in cognitive ability—the ability to think, reason, remember, and learn—that affects individuals' intellectual and social skills and interferes with their capacity to function in daily life. Severe cognitive difficulty is the core feature of dementia, but memory loss alone is not enough to diagnose it. In fact, memory loss may or may not be the most prominent feature of dementia. An individual diagnosed with dementia shows signs of impairment or decline in at least two areas of cognitive ability, shown in table 3.1, and this impairment must be severe enough to affect how the person functions socially and in daily living.

Recognizing impairment may be easier in some areas of cognitive ability than in others for family members of a person with declines in mental ability. In particular, the impairment of executive functions,

Table 3.1. Criteria for Diagnosing Dementia

Area of cognitive ability	Impairment	Example behaviors
Memory	Has difficulty recalling information from memory or learning new information	Can't remember something just heard; can't understand new information
Language	Has difficulty using language to communicate	Can't find the words needed; mixes up sentence structure so words come out in the wrong order; garbles speech
Motor skills	Has difficulty with coordination and carrying out motor activities	"Forgets" how to dance or ride a bike; has trouble dressing
Object recognition	Has difficulty recognizing or identifying objects	Doesn't recognize familiar faces; gets lost in familiar neighborhoods
Executive function	Has difficulty planning and organizing	See table 3.2

Source: Adapted from the American Psychiatric Association, *Diagnostic and Statistical Manual of Mental Disorders,* 4th ed., DSM-IV-TR (2000), www.mental-health-today .com/dep/dsm.htm.

Table 3.2. Features of Executive Dysfunction

Function	Description and examples
Insight	Is not aware of his memory problem
Judgment	Puts items in unusual places, such as milk into the cupboard instead of the refrigerator
Impulse control	Makes overly critical comments; drives aggressively
Problem-solving skills	Can no longer operate appliances, such as setting a timer on the oven, or do tasks he used to be able to do, like changing a car's tire
Social graces	Makes insensitive or inappropriate comments and jokes, uncharacteristic to his nature
Empathy	Is unconcerned about others' feelings; can't see a situation from their perspective
Initiative	Needs direction or assistance from others to do an activity; is uninterested in new activities and appears apathetic
Organization and planning	Has difficulty organizing and prioritizing pieces of information; can't figure out the steps needed to make an event happen
Multitasking	Can't do simultaneous activities, such as talking on the phone while cooking
Self-perception	Views situations selfishly and doesn't notice others' needs
Patience	Wants immediate gratification and is intolerant of inconveniences, such as waiting in line at a store

Source: R. Elliott, "Executive Functions and Their Disorders," *British Medical Bulletin* 65, no. 1 (2003):49–59.

called executive dysfunction, is often subtle and not easily detected early on. When you know what you're looking for, however, it can be easier to recognize. Executive function often changes gradually, with the impaired behaviors occurring sporadically. Family members frequently misattribute the behaviors as deliberate actions and will often complain that their loved one "has turned mean," "has become hostile," "won't cooperate anymore," "refuses to understand what I am saying," or "has fallen out of love with me." Table 3.2 presents features and examples of executive dysfunction (note that an individual may display only one or a few of these dysfunctions). Beyond recognizing executive dysfunction, family members and caregivers can also learn better ways to respond or cope with this impairment in their loved one; we discuss these strategies later in this chapter.

A person with dementia may exhibit a wide range of symptoms and behaviors, including

- depression
- anxiety
- agitation
- hallucinations
- paranoia
- delusions or false beliefs, such as accusing a spouse of having an affair
- oppositional behavior, such as refusing to bathe or change clothes
- wandering
- physical or verbal aggressiveness
- apathy

Alzheimer Disease

Alzheimer disease (AD) accounts for the illness experienced by about two-thirds of all individuals who suffer a dementia and typically appears in a person's 70s. Early-onset AD, however, can occur in individuals as early as their late 30s, and it is now known that these people have one or more genetic mutations, likely transmitted within families. Genetic factors also seem to contribute to AD that begins in later life, which is the more usual time for the disease to appear, but the way in which it is inherited is less clear. Later life AD is described as the sporadic variety of the disease.

Alzheimer disease is diagnosed on the basis of the individual displaying a gradual onset and continuing decline in memory loss and at least one of the other impairments in table 3.1. People with AD often show evidence of executive dysfunction before any memory changes occur, but as already mentioned, these signs are often overlooked or attributed to something else. AD typically progresses over 10 to 15 years, although the disease advances more rapidly in some individuals.

Scientists still don't know what triggers the disease to begin, but one of the characteristics of AD is the formation of structures in the brain called plaques and tangles. Plaques contain clumps of beta-amyloid protein, and tangles contain fibers of tau protein. Plaques and tangles are the structures that Alois Alzheimer, the physician who identified the disease, discovered in a deceased patient's brain in 1901. They distort the normal brain structure and function and lead to the death of brain cells, or neurons. The brain contains about 20 billion interconnected neurons, so losing a few makes no difference. When enough plaques or tangles accumulate, however, they can represent hundreds of thousands or millions of damaged neurons, which results in a noticeable loss of memory and other signs of cognitive impairment.

A definite diagnosis of AD can only be made by a pathologist examining a thin slice of brain tissue under a microscope for the presence of plaques and tangles. At the moment, the biopsy procedure to obtain brain tissue is too invasive and is done only for confirmation at autopsy. In the future, it may be possible to make a definitive diagnosis using noninvasive brain imaging scans combined with special markers injected into the bloodstream that "light up" the plaques and tangles or by detecting a biological marker in a blood sample.

Vascular Dementia

The second most common cause of dementia (10–15% of cases) is cerebrovascular disease. Vascular refers to the blood vessels, so in this disease, some of the arteries leading to the brain become narrowed or clogged so that blood flow is either restricted or stopped altogether to one or more parts of the brain. The arteries usually become narrowed due to atherosclerosis, which is a buildup of waxlike deposits, or plaque, inside arteries. Over time, the plaque can lead to damage of the artery walls and increase the chances of blood clots forming. A blocked artery feeding the heart causes a heart attack, while a blocked artery feeding the brain causes a stroke.

With a stroke, the diameter of the blocked artery dictates how much of the brain is damaged from receiving inadequate blood flow. To use the analogy of a tree, a major stroke would be a blockage in a large tree branch, and a minor stroke would be a blockage in a twig. Vascular dementia can result from either a few large strokes or an accumulation of minor strokes, in which hundreds or even thousands of tiny arteries become blocked. Both scenarios can damage the networks of nerve cells and cause deficits in memory or other brain functions.

In vascular dementia, the symptoms often progress steplike, with a plateau between each decline; each new stroke causes additional deficits. People with vascular dementia tend to be more emotional than people with AD, swinging from happy to sad from one moment to the next. Impairment of movement, such as muscle weakness and uncoordinated walking, are also more commonly seen in vascular dementia. Individuals with cerebrovascular disease often have vascular disease in other areas of their body as well, since atherosclerosis occurs throughout the entire body. For example, people with vascular dementia may have a history of heart attacks (cardiovascular disease) and blocked circulation to the legs (peripheral vascular disease). Depression is also a common feature of vascular dementia, as the same disease process also damages mood-sustaining circuitry within the brain.

Diffuse Lewy Body Dementia

Diffuse Lewy body dementia, or DLB, is named for Frederic Lewy, a physician who discovered abnormal clumps of proteins in the brain— Lewy bodies—that differ from plaques and tangles. Up to 10 percent of dementias have been diagnosed as DLB in the past, although recent research has shown that as many as 30 percent may actually be DLB dementia. DLB is a progressive dementia like Alzheimer disease.

People with DLB often exhibit a mixture of symptoms similar to Parkinson disease, including tremors, rigid muscles, walking with a broad gait, and having a flat facial expression, along with memory loss. People with DLB often experience peculiar visual hallucinations of people or animals, which can be vivid enough that the person tries to touch them. A person with DLB typically sees these hallucinations as curious or puzzling, sometimes friendly, and rarely frightening. Accompanying declines in intellectual ability allow the person to accept these hallucinations and not question their origins. For example, an individual with DLB might say, "I don't know why they come or how they get in here, but I see three little girls on the couch on most afternoons." Antipsychotic drugs can be effective at diminishing the intensity of disturbing visual hallucinations, but they must be given with care, because people with DLB can be very sensitive to the side effects of antipsychotic medications.

Fronto-temporal Dementia

About 10 percent of people with dementia have a form called fronto-temporal dementia, or FTD, which is due to nerve degeneration predominantly in the front (frontal lobe) and sides (temporal lobes) of the brain. Why the degeneration occurs is not well understood, although the most common cause of FTD is Pick's disease, which appears to be a genetic disorder that causes degeneration of brain tissue. Pick's disease runs in families and can show up as early as age 40 but, on average, appears in the mid-50s.

The damage from FTD impairs parts of the brain that normally control executive functions, the higher intellectual functions of planning, insight, judgment, and complex problem solving. People with FTD show prominent executive dysfunction early on, with personality changes, and they have less memory impairment until the later stages of the disease. A special brain imaging test called positron emission tomography, or PET, is used to diagnose this disorder.

Other Causes of Dementia

Other causes of dementia include various degenerative diseases, such as Parkinson disease, multiple sclerosis, and Huntington disease. These diseases cause degeneration of various parts of the brain, which can affect memory and other brain functions as well as movement.

Some infections also target the brain and can leave lasting damage that leads to dementia, including severe meningitis, late stage syphilis, HIV infection, and various other infectious agents.

Chronic alcoholism can cause permanent brain damage, predominantly exhibited as uncoordinated movements and short-term memory problems of an unusual type, called confabulation, where the person imagines and believes detailed stories that are not true. This form of dementia is termed alcoholic dementia. Lack of vitamin B1 (thiamine) is key to the brain damage from chronic alcoholism, so replacing thiamine can sometimes, but not always, improve memory function.

Any condition that disrupts the supply of oxygen or glucose to the brain for a period can lead to permanent brain damage. For example, people who have survived a heart attack where the heartbeat stopped for more than a few minutes, those who have been overcome by carbon monoxide (most often due to a faulty home furnace), and those with severe diabetes who have a prolonged period of low blood sugar can all develop symptoms of dementia.

Boxers frequently develop a type of dementia called dementia pugilistica from repeated blows to the head. Each blow causes microscopic tearing of tiny blood vessels under the skull, and the accumulation of thousands of blows can lead to permanent dementia. Repeated concussions in athletes playing other contact sports, such as football, can also result in this type of dementia.

Mild Cognitive Impairment

Mild cognitive impairment, or MCI, is the diagnosis made in individuals who display some impairment of memory or the other cognitive functions listed in table 3.1, but the impairments are not severe enough to be considered dementia. In other words, these individuals can still function in their daily lives, especially if they use tools like establishing routines and using a day planner or calendar. Since people don't transform overnight from having normal brain function to meeting the criteria for dementia, a diagnosis of MCI includes those in the early stages of developing Alzheimer disease and other dementias. Not all individuals with MCI progress over time to a diagnosis of dementia, however, which reflects the limitations of current diagnostic tools and techniques at making accurate predictions.

MCI is further subdivided for individuals with primarily memory complaints and those with other cognitive impairments, such as executive dysfunction. Every year, 12.5 to 15 percent of people with the memory impairment form of MCI progress to a diagnosis of Alzheimer disease.

Diagnosing Dementia

A medical evaluation for dementia—the so-called dementia workup— typically includes a series of blood tests, which are done to try to find a reason for the person's complaints about memory or other brain function problems. Brain imaging scans and other specialized testing may also be performed; however, the diagnosis of dementia is still largely based on signs (evidence of the disease observed by a physician) and symptoms (evidence of the disease reported by the patient). Table 3.3 lists possible tests and their purpose.

Table 3.3. Tests to Evaluate for Causes of Dementia

Test	Purpose
Blood tests	
Complete blood count	Detects infections; detects anemia (low number of red blood cells or low hemoglobin in the blood, both of which indicate that the blood can't carry enough oxygen)
Vitamin B12	Determines B12 concentration; adequate B12 is essential for forming blood cells and for brain and nerve function
Thyroid	Determines whether the thyroid hormone level is too high (hyperthyroidism) or too low (hypothyroidism)
Electrolytes	Determines the concentration of minerals, such as sodium, potassium, and calcium; mineral levels must remain within narrow limits for good nerve and brain function
Specialized blood tests	Detects other infectious agents, such as those that cause AIDS, syphilis, and meningitis
Other tests	
Electroencephalogram (EEG)	Detects problems in the brain's electrical activity; EEG can help to diagnose seizure and delirium (acute brain failure due to a medical condition such as a severe infection)
Brain imaging, such as magnetic resonance imaging (MRI), computerized axial tomography (CAT scan), or positron emission tomography (PET)	Detects evidence of strokes, tumors, malformations, or atrophy (tissue wasting or shrinkage)
Neuropsychological testing, or "paper and pencil" tests	Assesses various brain function abilities, such as memory, language, calculation ability, and problem-solving skills; a neuropsychologist administers various possible tests and compares the results to norms for age and education, and primary care physicians commonly use screening tests such as the mini mental status exam (MMSE) and the Montreal cognitive assessment (MoCA)

When Dementia and Depression Occur Together

Depression occurs in about half of all people with dementia for various reasons. As dementia damages brain tissue, some of the areas affected are those involved in sustaining mood. Some people with AD are aware of their declining memory and become distressed or depressed by it. Dementia victims often eat poorly as well, which puts them at further risk of poor brain function and greater risk of depression. Severe depression can also herald the onset of a rapid cognitive decline into dementia.

The symptoms of depression in a person with dementia can be identical to the symptoms in a cognitively normal person; however, the depressive symptoms may make the dementia appear to be further progressed than it actually is. Therefore, when an individual has depression with what looks like dementia, the ideal course is to try to treat the depression adequately first. With the depression "removed," a physician can see the true nature of the cognitive impairment and treat it accordingly. Often times, the person's cognition improves dramatically once the depression has been treated, but at other times, the change is only minor.

There is some evidence of a possible link between depression and the risk of developing dementia. The hippocampus, a seahorse-shaped part of the brain, is very sensitive to damage from repeated episodes of depression. MRI (magnetic resonance imaging) scans have actually been able to show the hippocampus shrink with depression and "regrow" with adequate treatment. This part of the brain is also critical in memory processing and is one of the first areas to show deteriorating function in Alzheimer disease. Although the possibility of depression leading to dementia is still unproven, the current evidence argues for getting treatment for depression to prevent this possible risk factor link.

Risk Factors for Dementia

Although it's normal for the memory to slow down to a mild degree as a person gets older, aging is not a cause of the severe impairments that lead to dementia. Thousands of individuals live through their 80s, 90s, and beyond with an intact and sharp memory. Nevertheless, the proportion of the population with a memory disorder does increase with age; for example, more people in their 80s have Alzheimer disease than people in their 60s.

People with a genetic family history of dementia are at greater risk of developing dementia themselves, although again, it's not a given. For example, many people have family members with dementia but do not themselves develop symptoms of impaired brain function, and many people with dementia have no family history of the illness. Some gene mutations are known to increase the risk of developing Alzheimer disease and other forms of dementia, such as the mutation that causes Huntington disease.

Brain injury is a risk factor for developing both Alzheimer disease and dementia pugilistica, although there may be different mechanisms involved. One may be that the brain repairs the injury in the manner of a bricklayer repairing a damaged brick wall by placing bricks haphazardly instead of in a highly ordered pattern.

Current research points to multiple pathways that can lead to AD, with some of the known risk factors being

- family history of AD in first-degree relatives (parents or siblings)
- hypothyroidism
- history of traumatic brain injury
- possibly repeat episodes of depression

Risk factors for vascular dementia include any condition that increases the chances of atherosclerosis, or deposits in the arteries, and therefore the potential for stroke. Minor restrictions to blood flow to the brain can cause temporary visual defects, impaired speech, and weakness or numbness that often resolve on their own. These temporary events are known as transient ischemic attacks, or TIAs, and are an indicator of possible atherosclerosis in blood vessels feeding the brain. People at greatest risk for developing atherosclerosis include those who have

- diabetes mellitus (either type 1 or type 2)
- high blood pressure
- high levels of "bad" cholesterol, which is a lipid called low-density lipoprotein (LDL), in the blood

- an irregular heart rate, which can cause a blood clot to form in the heart and then be carried elsewhere, such as the brain, where it blocks an artery (atrial fibrillation)
- cardiovascular or peripheral vascular disease
- a history of smoking
- a family history of atherosclerosis

The main risk factor for diffuse Lewy body and fronto-temporal dementias is currently thought to be a family history of these dementias.

Treatment and Management

As we mentioned earlier, memory loss and impairments to other brain functions can be the result of potentially reversible conditions. For example, if vitamin B12 deficiency, low levels of thyroid hormone, or medication side effects are the cause of cognitive impairment, then addressing that cause can improve or restore brain function. In this section, however, we focus on treatment options for people diagnosed with irreversible dementia.

There is no cure for AD or other progressive dementias, although researchers are looking into possibilities for a vaccine or other technique that could prevent plaque formation and therefore stop the disease from progressing. Another key to better treatment of this disease would be to detect it early enough to mount effective interventions to slow its course or even to block its cumulative deleterious effects. For this reason, one avenue of AD research is investigating reliable markers in blood samples or on brain imaging scans that would allow a definite diagnosis to be made at a very early stage in the disease's onset.

At the moment, however, the treatment options include a few medications that can slow the progression of AD and possibly other dementias. In addition, symptoms and behaviors related to dementia can be treated with medications, such as antidepressants, sedatives, or antipsychotic drugs in appropriately small doses. Certain factors that contribute to dementia, specifically the risk factors involved in atherosclerosis, can also be modified with anticoagulant medications to reduce the formation of more blood clots.

Treatments for Alzheimer Disease

Two types of medication are currently available to slow the progression of Alzheimer disease and other progressive dementias.

1. Cholinesterase inhibitors or cholinegeric enhancers. The three available cholinesterase inhibitors are donepezil (brand name Aricept), galantamine (Nivalin, Razadyne, Razadyne ER, Reminyl, Lycoremine), and rivastigmine (Exelon). These drugs slow down the degradation of a chemical called acetylcholine, which is a neurotransmitter, or chemical messenger, that mainly assists with thinking and learning. The predominant damage from the brain plaques seen in AD is to the brain cells that contain acetylcholine. Therefore, these drugs boost the acetylcholine levels within the damaged (but not yet dead) brain cells, thus enhancing their ability to communicate with each other. Increasing acetylcholine levels has no effect on dead brain cells, so the drugs can't stop AD but can merely delay its increasing severity.

About one-third of people with mild to moderate Alzheimer disease report that these medications noticeably improve their memory, and family members often report increases in an individual's alertness, social interaction, and ability to carry out everyday tasks. These medications do not stop the disease process, however; they merely slow it down for a time. Nevertheless, this delay might provide two more years with good quality of life or postpone nursing home placement with its associated high costs.

Common side effects of these medications are nausea, vomiting, stomach pain, constipation or diarrhea, nightmares, and sometimes headaches.

2. Memantine (brand name Namenda). Memantine blocks the toxic effect of another neurotransmitter, called glutamate. Although glutamate is necessary for brain function, there seems to be an imbalance in people with Alzheimer disease. The connection between glutamate and AD is not well understood, but memantine has demonstrated modest benefits on cognitive function, similar to the benefits of cholinesterase inhibitors. Potential side effects of memantine include dizziness, confusion, headache, and constipation.

The current standard treatment for AD is to combine these two medications to try to slow the progression of symptoms as much as possible. Currently, the FDA has approved these drugs for people with a diagnosis of dementia but not for mild cognitive impairment. Both drugs are costly, and the cost may be prohibitive for people with limited insurance coverage. Medicare and Medicaid provide coverage for these medications. If depression coexists with AD, then the individual may need to be treated with an antidepressant and an AD medication at the same time.

Psychotherapy is not traditionally used to treat people with a memory problem because impaired recall has been thought to impede progress from one session to the next. Recent research suggests, however, that modified counseling techniques can be successful in helping address an individual's thoughts and feelings about his illness, its associated symptoms, and the problems that result from having AD. Interpersonal psychotherapy, which involves simultaneous counseling for both the person with AD and his caregivers or family members, can also be an effective way for everyone involved to better understand the illness and be part of the treatment process.

Treatments for Vascular Dementia

Treatment of vascular dementia aims to prevent the individual from having more strokes, thus minimizing the chances of further cognitive decline. Because blood clots can form in the arteries damaged by atherosclerosis (plaque buildup and damage to the artery wall) and cause more strokes, treatment involves controlling as many of the risk factors for atherosclerosis and blood clots as possible (see "Risk Factors for Dementia," earlier in this chapter).

Aspirin decreases the stickiness of platelets (the cells in the blood involved in clotting) and is commonly used to reduce the tendency of clots to form. Aspirin can produce other problems, however, including an increased risk of bleeding from ulcers. Anticoagulants, or blood thinners, are also used to prevent blood clots. Sometimes, blood tests are required to ensure that the reduction in clotting tendency does not go too far and increase the risk of bleeding too easily. People who take anticoagulants need to be extra careful to avoid cuts or injuries, as bleeding can be more severe. These drugs must be stopped or reversed by other means prior to elective surgery as well.

Vascular blockage in the carotid arteries, which are the main feeder arteries to the brain, can sometimes be located using ultrasound or other imaging techniques. In the case of a serious blockage (greater than 70% obstructed), the artery can be reopened with specialized techniques or through surgery. These techniques can restore good blood flow and reduce the risk of another clot completely restricting the artery, which would cause a major stroke. Smaller arteries cannot be reopened by these methods, so drug intervention to reduce the tendency to form clots is the only treatment option, along with reducing the risk factors for atherosclerosis.

Treatments for DLB, FTD, and Other Dementias

Other progressive dementias, such as diffuse Lewy body dementia, may also benefit from the treatments already described for Alzheimer disease. Otherwise, current treatment for dementia involves managing symptoms and difficulties that arise from the illness, including depression, anxiety, agitation, paranoia, delusions, oppositional behavior, aggressiveness, and others. Various medications can limit the severity of these symptoms, and family members and caregivers can learn strategies for coping with them. Sometimes, the burden on family members is too great and a nursing home with round-the-clock assistance is needed to provide dignified and safe care. We discuss nursing homes and other care facilities in chapter 11.

Herbal Preparations

As we discussed in chapter 1, herbal preparations and other supplements don't undergo rigorous testing and aren't regulated by the FDA. Claims about their effectiveness tend to be based on anecdotal reports. Rigorous scientific proof of effectiveness is lacking, although this fact does not seem to slow the sale of these items. Several preparations are advertised as having benefits for preserving brain function or slowing the progression of dementia, including

- vitamin E, which some reports suggest can slow the progression of AD; In high doses, vitamin E can be toxic and can cause increased bleeding for people with stomach ulcers
- antioxidants, which have been linked with various health benefits, including the prevention of dementia; they are found in the so-called super foods, such as blueberries
- *Gingko biloba* extracts, which have been claimed to have anti-

oxidant properties; however, a recent rigorous study found no measurable prevention of memory loss

- Omega-3 fatty acids, which may reduce the risk of various diseases, including dementia; they are found in fish oil and some other foods

Check with your primary care doctor before adding these substances to your diet.

Living with Dementia

Because many dementias are progressive and treatment does not stop the disease process, many people with dementia and their family members feel condemned when the diagnosis is made. In the case of Alzheimer disease, the most common dementia, early evaluation and intervention with the currently available treatments do offer moderate benefits by slowing its progression. Nevertheless, the implications of dementia for individuals and their family members include the potential for significant dependence, emotional strain, time commitments, and financial costs, as well as changing roles in the family. The people who cope best are those who already have a balanced, healthy, and stimulating lifestyle; an adequate support system; stable housing arrangements; and access to quality medical and psychiatric care.

Finding out as much as possible about dementia and its implications is an important first step for the person receiving a diagnosis and for the person taking on the role of caregiver. Several good books and websites give details about caring for a person with dementia as the condition progresses. Some of these resources are listed at the back of this book. Here, we describe briefly some key points for people diagnosed with dementia and their caregivers to consider.

In early stages, the person may be able to continue living independently with some help from family members or friends, but as the condition progresses, more constant care becomes necessary. In later stages, the individual may need a nurse or nursing home care. This situation might not occur until 10 to 15 years after the initial diagnosis, although the disease progresses more rapidly in some people, for reasons that are poorly understood.

People with dementia may face, and eventually need help with, the following tasks and behaviors:

- Getting adequate nutrition. As well as losing interest in food, people in the later stages of dementia can lose control of muscles used for chewing and swallowing and therefore more easily choke or inhale food into the lungs.
- Taking medications, both at the correct time and at the right dose.
- Dealing with finances, home maintenance, appointments, medical decisions, and similar tasks.
- Staying safe while doing activities that require problem-solving skills. For example, daily activities like cooking, driving, or even walking down the street may present challenges that a person with dementia has difficulty negotiating safely.
- Communicating. As well as affecting how well individuals can tell caregivers what they need or want, difficulty communicating can lead to isolation and depression.
- Coping with their emotions. While some behaviors may stem from impaired brain functions, others may be the result of trying to cope with their dementia symptoms. For example, dementia can lead to aggression, confusion, depression, and anxiety.
- Getting adequate sleep. People with dementia often experience sleep problems, like insomnia, wandering at night, and day/night reversal.
- Maintaining basic hygiene, including bathing, dressing, and using the toilet.

Personality change can be an acutely difficult feature of dementia, particularly for a caregiving spouse. Spouses typically say things like, "He's not the man I married," "She's lost in her own world and doesn't seem to care about me anymore," or "He's not dead, but he's already gone for me." These experiences can cause the caregiver to feel grief, as well as other emotions ranging from compassion and altruism to anger, resentment, and even hostility. Many family members have described loved ones with AD and other dementias as having occasional good days, when they recall old memories and show a flicker of their former personality. Equally common are bad days, when all functions are worse than usual.

Problem behaviors, such as hallucinations, delusions, wandering, and repetitive vocalizations, can also be distressing, both for the individual with dementia and for caregivers. Books dedicated to discussing AD and other dementias, and organizations that provide support for people and families dealing with dementia, offer ideas and guidance about coping with problem behaviors. Some of these sources are listed in the resources section at the end of this book.

People with dementia show varying degrees of insight into their cognitive decline. Some may be completely unaware of it and deny that they have a problem, even when confronted with evidence. Insisting that people with dementia "admit" they can no longer perform a particular task is often futile, because brain impairments decrease the ability to grasp the big picture. Other people with dementia do realize that they are losing their memory and other cognitive abilities and can become quite distressed and depressed as a result. For these individuals, it is sometimes helpful to ease their guilt or self-blame by reminding them that their cognitive impairment is due to an underlying brain disease not under their control and not due to a character flaw.

Once Alzheimer disease and other dementias progress past a certain point, afflicted people tend to lose insight into their impairments and stop comparing their current and prior lives. They no longer fret as much about what they have lost and can actually seem happier and more content. They seem to live more in the moment, becoming preoccupied with their present activity. This stage of dementia can ease some of the caregiver burden, since the caregiver can create a schedule of activities to occupy the person. Adult daycare centers provide such structured activities and other services for people with dementia and allow caregivers to take a break and tend to their own needs.

Keeping Your Brain Healthy

Maintaining a lifestyle that promotes brain health makes sense:

- Eat a healthy diet that incorporates a variety of foods, including generous amounts of fresh fruits and vegetables.
- Exercise your brain. Studies have shown that people in their 60s

and older can slow cognitive decline by regularly reading about current events, doing crossword puzzles, and participating in mind-stimulating games or other intellectual pursuits.

- Protect your brain in the literal sense. Use a seat belt while driving, make sure your vehicle's airbags work properly, and wear protective headgear for sports like bicycling, motorcycling, skiing, and skydiving.
- Reduce alcohol consumption (see chapter 8). Excess intake can cause permanent brain damage, particularly to memory, judgment, and motor coordination.
- Get physical exercise and be socially active.
- Get enough sleep.

■ ■ ■

If You Are Concerned about Your Memory or Other Brain Functions

- Learn as much as you can about memory loss and dementia.
- Talk with a family member, trusted friend, or someone you respect in your community.
- Make an appointment to see your primary care doctor.
- Stay as physically active as possible.
- Participate in social activities.
- Join a support group or participate in an online community for people with memory loss.
- Ask someone you trust to help you with important decisions.

Suggestions for Family Members and Caregivers

Caregivers who live with a person with dementia often become so preoccupied by caring for their loved one that they neglect their own needs. They have higher rates of depression, are more likely to abuse alcohol or other substances, and have poorer health than the general population. Given the situations that caregivers often face— questions repeated over and over, their loved one wandering out the door and becoming lost, obstinate behaviors like refusing to shower or change clothes, accusations of infidelity, or even threats of violence—it is no surprise that they can experience distress themselves.

Adult children often provide a great deal of help but commonly feel frustrated by poor cooperation from the person with dementia, geographic distance, competing duties such as their job or childcare, and the discomfort of recognizing the role reversal with their parent.

Here are a few suggestions if you are facing a new role as caregiver for a person with dementia:

- Find a source of practical advice and support. Many books, support groups, and organizations are available, some of which are listed in the resources.
- Phone a local geriatric center. Many centers have social workers to work closely with caregivers and help them access community services. They can also help find suitable nursing home placement should that become necessary.
- Be supportive of the person with dementia. Talk with and listen to him. Reassure him that life can still be enjoyed.
- Offer your help with tasks that require problem solving or making decisions.
- Take care of yourself. Don't feel shy about asking for help when you need it, and take time away regularly to rest, do personal errands, meet with a friend, or just be relieved of responsibility for a while. Taking care of your own emotional and physical health will help you care for your loved one better and be able to sustain the effort long term.

FOUR

Living with Illness and Disability

In 1900, the mean life expectancy in America was 50 years. By 2000, it had risen to 80 years. This immense increase has been due to numerous medical and social advances, including lower infant mortality, improved sanitation systems, vaccination programs, early cancer detection, and improvements in both medications and procedures to treat many medical conditions. Although Americans are living longer, however, many are doing so with an accumulation of chronic medical problems, hearing and vision deficits, and dementia.

Today's 65-year-old can look forward to 15 or more years of retirement, yet many aging Americans fear that their savings will be inadequate to pay for health care over the remainder of their lives. Along with these fears, add chronic pain, limited mobility, and a list of prescribed medications, among other issues, and it's understandable how medical problems and their treatment can often create anxiety and depression.

Some medical illnesses themselves cause depression or anxiety, and suffering from anxiety or depression can worsen the perception of illness severity, pain intensity, or associated disability. Chronic diseases such as congestive heart failure, emphysema, Parkinson disease, and Alzheimer disease commonly have depression associated with them. As well as amplifying the illness symptoms and pain intensity, the depression can undermine compliance with treatment and lead to shortened life expectancy.

Anxiety can accompany depression in the face of medical illness as individuals worry about not being able to meet their responsibilities or to enjoy life as they used to. Treatment of anxiety and depression along with treatment of the underlying condition simultaneously can help maintain independence and result in better quality of life.

In this chapter, we include information about illnesses and prescription drugs that are commonly associated with depression. We describe in more detail four types of illness—arthritis, stroke, heart disease, and cancer—that older people often encounter and how depression can interact with these illnesses. We also discuss disabilities that can limit mobility and independence.

Chronic Illness and Depression

In some instances, depressive symptoms can be the direct result of a chronic illness. For example, some cancers, such as pancreatic cancer, can produce chemicals that circulate in the bloodstream and affect the brain, leading to depression. Diseases that affect the central nervous system, including Parkinson disease, Alzheimer disease, and multiple sclerosis, can cause depression by interfering with or damaging mood-sustaining circuits within the brain. Damage to the brain's mood circuitry can also occur after a large stroke that chokes off the blood supply to one or more areas of the brain or after an accumulation of small strokes, which commonly happens in people with chronically high blood pressure or diabetes.

Other medical conditions are risk factors for depression, because the illness's symptoms or limitations lead to depression. For example, having heart or lung disease that is severe enough to limit a person's exercise tolerance can cause depression because it restricts independence. Chronic pain is a well-known risk factor, because it is distressing to be in pain all the time, particularly if it restricts a person's activity, constantly intrudes on her consciousness, or disrupts a good night's sleep. We discuss chronic pain in more detail in chapter 5.

Some individuals experience depression as a side effect of various prescription drugs, as shown in table 4.1. Common culprits are drugs for high blood pressure, steroids, some anticancer drugs, and some immune system–regulation drugs used to treat diseases like multiple sclerosis and hepatitis C. The long-term use of narcotic pain medications, antianxiety medications, and sedatives can also predispose some individuals to depression.

Table 4.1. Prescription Drugs That May Cause Depression

Drug category	Conditions treated with the drugs	Examples
Antiviral	Shingles, herpes	Acyclovir (Zovirax)
Anticonvulsants	Epileptic seizures	Phenytoin (Dilantin)
Barbiturates	Anxiety, epileptic seizures	Phenobarbitol
Benzodiazepines	Anxiety, insomnia	Diazepam (Valium), Lorazepam (Ativan)
Beta-adrenergic blockers	High blood pressure, heart failure, other heart problems	Propranolol (Inderal)
Dopamine enhancers	Parkinson disease	Parlodel (Bromocriptine)
Calcium-channel blockers	High blood pressure, chest pain, congestive heart failure	Diltiazem (e.g., Cardiazem)
Metabolic blocker	Alcoholism	Disulfiram (Antabuse)
Hormones	Menopause, osteoporosis	Estrogen, progesterone
Certain antibiotics	Certain bacterial infections	Fluoroquinolones (e.g., Ciprofloxacin)
Statins	High cholesterol, coronary (heart) artery disease, heart attack prevention	Atorvastatin (Lipitor)
Immune regulators	Certain cancers, hepatitis B	Interferon alpha (Intron)
Narcotics	Intense pain	Oxycontin (Oxycodone), morphine

Source: WebMD, Drugs That Cause Depression (2005), www.webmd.com/depression/guide/medicines-cause-depression.

Common Chronic Illnesses as We Age
Arthritis

Arthritis is a disease in which joints become inflamed. Typical symptoms are pain, stiffness, swelling, and a decrease in the joint's range of motion. The most common form of arthritis is osteoarthritis, or "wear and tear" arthritis, which occurs when cartilage and other components of the joint are degraded or destroyed from years of use. Osteoarthritis can be exacerbated by the repetitive use of certain joints in work or play (repetitive motion injury) or from the added strain the joints take when a person is overweight or obese. A second common form of arthritis is rheumatoid arthritis, which is an autoimmune disorder, meaning that the body's own immune system attacks healthy tissue. With rheumatoid arthritis, the immune system attacks a part of the joint that contains lubricating fluid; over time, this can lead to destruction of both cartilage and bone in the joint. Risk factors for arthritis include family history, obesity, and earlier injury of a joint.

The body responds to the damaged tissue with an attempt to "clean up the mess" by mounting an inflammatory response that can lead to redness, swelling, and fluid accumulation within the joint space. Treatment with anti-inflammatory medications can be very helpful to control pain, swelling, and inflammation, although these medications do have the potentially serious side effects of bleeding, high blood pressure, and kidney damage. Sometimes, excess fluid can be withdrawn from the joint space with a needle to relieve pressure and reduce pain. Stronger anti-inflammatory agents, such as steroids and lubricating substances to mimic the effect of natural cartilage, can also be injected into the joint space. These strategies often work for some years, but as the joint damage continues, more deformity, pain, and limited movement can result. In some cases, surgical joint fusion or joint replacement may be options of last resort.

Severe arthritis can limit a person's mobility and can make it exceptionally difficult to perform daily tasks, especially if the arthritis is in the hand or arm joints. For many people, this situation becomes depressing as they become more and more dependent on other people to help them with daily living, and as their pain seems to take over their lives. We discuss pain management in chapter 5.

Stroke and Heart Attack

Strokes and heart attacks occur for the same basic reason—lack of blood flow to a particular organ—but in different parts of the body. A stroke involves the blockage or rupture of an artery feeding a part of the brain, while a heart attack involves a blockage to one of three major arteries feeding the heart.

With strokes, the larger an artery's diameter, the greater the damage. Some strokes are so tiny that people don't know they're having them until the effects of enough tiny strokes accumulate to produce inefficiencies in brain signals. The early signs of having suffered a stroke are

- suddenly having difficulty speaking or walking
- developing paralysis suddenly or over the course of several minutes to hours, or waking up with paralysis
- leaning to one side while walking
- suddenly losing vision in one eye or losing vision in part of the normal field of view
- losing the ability to move an arm or a leg, or an arm and a leg together on the same side of the body
- suddenly developing a severe headache
- suddenly developing confusion
- sudden onset of dizziness or vertigo (the sensation that the room is spinning)

A heart attack, medically called a myocardial infarction, results from a blockage in one of the coronary arteries that feeds the heart muscle. The main coronary arteries have three main branches, and, as with strokes, the larger the diameter of the blocked artery, the more heart muscle is deprived of oxygen. Sometimes, but not always, narrowed coronary arteries that cannot keep up with the heart's demand for adequate oxygen (during physical exertion, for example) produce symptoms of chest pain, called angina. This can be a warning signal that the heart is not getting enough oxygen-rich blood to function properly.

With both strokes and heart attacks, the artery usually becomes blocked by a blood clot that forms on the inside of the artery wall where it has been damaged by the buildup of deposits, called atherosclerotic plaque. The risk factors for forming plaque and therefore being more susceptible to having a stroke or heart attack are

- smoking
- high blood pressure
- a type of heartbeat disturbance called atrial fibrillation
- high cholesterol

- diabetes
- obesity
- family history of stroke or heart attack

Medications such as aspirin, warfarin (brand name Coumadin), or clopidogel (Plavix) can be taken in an attempt to prevent further blood clots. Regular use of these medications as well as reducing the risk factors listed above can help lower the risk of having another stroke or heart attack.

After a stroke, rehabilitation through intensive physical and speech therapy can retrain the parts of the brain not permanently damaged by the stroke and can sometimes improve the resulting acute paralysis, speech deficits, or dizziness. The brain has some ability to compensate for deficits—undamaged parts of the brain take over tasks previously performed by the now-damaged area. In some cases, functions can be restored to near normal. Even with rehabilitation, however, some people who have had one or more strokes may be left with varying degrees of paralysis, speech deficits, dizziness, visual field restrictions, difficulty concentrating, and other, more subtle mental changes.

Strokes are a well-known cause of depression for two reasons. The stroke itself can damage mood-sustaining circuits within the brain, while the physical or mental deficits that result from the stroke can precipitate depression or anxiety when people find they are less able or unable to do tasks and activities previously taken for granted.

After a heart attack, narrowed coronary arteries can be reopened with stents, which are metal tubes placed within the narrowed area to enlarge it and therefore restore blood flow. Surviving a heart attack is an eye-opening experience for most people. They often have a profound perception that their lives have been spared for the moment, and they frequently fear having another heart attack. They may also worry about resuming sports, vigorous exercise, and sexual activity. These feelings and concerns can provoke strong anxiety, depression, or both.

When people with heart disease—narrowing of the arteries supplying the heart—become depressed, it can be a fatal complication. The reason is uncertain, but it probably has to do with several factors. Fighting a serious illness can require every ounce of a person's inner strength, yet depression can undermine that fight. People who are depressed also tend to lack the willingness to be rigorous about taking medications on time as prescribed. Failing to take medications correctly can lead to continued high risk for heart attacks, strokes, or other complications, such as an abnormal heartbeat, congestive heart failure, or weakness of the heart muscle, which decreases its pumping potential.

Heart disease complications can also cause or worsen depression and anxiety. For example, congestive heart failure can lead to severely restricted exercise potential, even to the point of being limited to a few steps before feeling exhausted or short of breath. This situation can then lead to depression and anxiety, as even basic self-care becomes a great effort, and participation in life's activities, in general, is severely limited.

Complying with other health recommendations, such as altering dietary habits, losing weight, getting more rest, or cutting down alcohol consumption can all seem harder for a depressed person. The illness of depression itself can also produce changes in hormone levels and biorhythms that can further strain an already diseased body. Finally, depression can lead to suicidal thoughts and loss of the will to live any longer.

For people who are obese, eat a high-calorie or high-fat diet, smoke, don't exercise, have inadequately treated high blood pressure, or have inadequately controlled diabetes, even modest lifestyle changes can play a significant role in reducing the risk for further strokes or heart attacks.

Cancer

The term *cancer* encompasses so many different illnesses, with such a variety of symptoms, risk factors, and treatments, that we can't give these details here. One thing that these illnesses have in common, however, is that receiving a diagnosis of cancer strikes fear into most people. Cancer treatment can also be a taxing ordeal, especially chemotherapy, which is basically taking poisons that target fast-growing cells more than normal cells in the hope of killing the cancer cells but allowing the individual to survive the experience. Cancer treatment can continue for months or even years, which, in addition to the physical toll, can wear down a person's morale, especially if she doesn't have a strong support system. A positive mental attitude affects the success of cancer treatment.

About one-quarter of people with cancer also have depression, but it can be difficult to recognize symptoms as depression, since fatigue, sleep disturbances, and other symptoms may also be the result of the cancer itself or the treatment. As with anyone experiencing these and other symptoms of depression, however, if they last for two weeks or longer, the individual should be evaluated for depression. Diagnosing and properly treating the disorder is critical to individuals' chances of successfully undergoing their cancer treatment, as well as improving quality of life.

A relatively new method of fighting cancer by manipulating the immune system shows a lot of promise, but it is frequently accompanied by depression. For example, people treated with interferon—proteins made naturally by cells in the immune system—show a 50 percent incidence of severe depression as a side effect of the treatment. Some treatment centers pretreat their patients with antidepressants in anticipation.

Coping with Disability from Illness or Accident

Jean was age 62, married with three grown children, and still teaching high school when she was diagnosed with multiple sclerosis. Her symptoms began with losing vision in her left eye. Her walking became uncoordinated, and she seemed to list toward one side. On two occasions she would have fallen had her husband not been at her side.

After the initial shock of the diagnosis and a period of what she called "feeling sorry for myself," Jean decided to be proactive in dealing with her illness. She took her medications faithfully, followed up regularly with her neurologist and primary care physician, and began an exercise program at a nearby gym, with a personal trainer to develop a program for her.

Despite these measures, Jean had some setbacks. She had two flare-ups, with further loss of motor function, this time in her left leg. These setbacks upset her. At about the same time, her mother developed a series of medical problems, and Jean, her sister, and her brother decided to place their mother in a nursing home. Of the three siblings, Jean was the only one living in the same city as their mother, so she felt responsible for watching over her mother. A short while later, Jean's eld-est daughter announced her engagement to be married the following spring. Jean's joy quickly turned to nervousness and panicky anxiety, be-cause she wanted to help prepare for the wedding but feared that the stress would cause another flare-up of her MS.

At her next appointment, Jean's neurologist started her on an anti-depressant and suggested that she see a psychiatrist as well to help her cope better emotionally. The psychiatrist helped Jean brainstorm some ideas for managing the demands in her life that were increasing her stress. Jean identified three things that seemed to trigger a relapse of her MS:

1. Letting herself get too tired. She found that a one-hour afternoon nap really helped her stamina, but she often didn't take time for a nap.
2. Getting too warm. (People with MS are often sensitive to heat and feel weaker in hot climates or even after taking a hot bath.)
3. Feeling stressed from too many obligations. She said she often had a sinking feeling of never being able to catch up. In addition to continuing to teach full time, she sponsored an extracurricular debate club at the school, was active on church committees, and attended two different book clubs.

With the help of her psychiatrist, Jean came to understand that she couldn't expect herself to multitask as easily as she used to because she now had to contend with a degenerative neurological illness. Jean's psychiatrist suggested that she think of her daily allotment of energy as a pie chart in which certain things were essential (eating, bathing, cooking, sleeping, etc.). He then asked her to rank her usual "nonessen-tial" activities from most to least important, to think about the energy each one cost her, and to decide which ones could fit into the remaining energy in her pie chart.

When confronted with this black-and-white assessment, Jean real-ized that she was clearly trying to do too much, especially since she now considered her daily workouts and afternoon naps to be essentials in her pie chart. Jean decided it was time to make some changes to lessen her sense of being overloaded. She eventually decided to withdraw from one book club, ask a fellow teacher to assume the debate club sponsor-

ship after the current year ended, ask her brother to take responsibility
for overseeing their mother's finances, and hire a professional wedding
coordinator to help with her daughter's wedding planning.

With her psychiatrist's help, Jean came to terms with the fact that
her illness would flare up if she overcommitted herself. She successfully
kept to her lighter schedule and had no further relapses leading up to
her daughter's wedding.

With many diseases that become more common with age, people
experience physical limitations as a complication of the disease process. In other instances, accidents cause sudden limits to mobility
and independence. People who become permanently disabled from
whatever cause frequently experience anxiety early on, and depression often follows when the reality of their new situation sinks in. In
severe cases, the risk of suicide can increase.

The relationship between depression and disability goes in both
directions; that is, disability can lead to depression, and depression
can lead to further disability. For example, if people with emphysema (a lung disease that causes shortness of breath), congestive heart
failure, or Parkinson disease become depressed from the disability
associated with their chronic illness, the combination of the physical
illness plus the depression makes them significantly more disabled
overall. Conversely, successfully relieving the depression lightens the
total load of physical disability plus depression, even if the underlying chronic medical condition does not change.

People who are able to adjust to the demands of their disabilities
by successfully making accommodations to lifestyle and accepting
these accommodations as reasonable and practical can decrease the
risk of further depression. Accommodations may include having a
wheelchair, access ramps, an adapted automobile, and other assis-
tive devices. Hiring a paid caregiver or moving into an assisted living
facility may also be necessary, especially if family members don't live
close enough or aren't willing to offer assistance. Senior apartment
complexes and other facilities anticipate the needs of aging individuals through building design, with easy access by foot and wheelchair,
elevators, common areas for social interaction, alarm systems such as
pull-strings to summon help if needed, and security systems. Some
apartment complexes offer hot meal programs within the building at

a reasonable cost, and many facilities offer some form of regular bus or van service to get to doctor visits or to go shopping.

Driving

Driving is a complex act that requires the fluid coordination of several body systems, including vision, hearing, cognitive processing, reflexes, and flexibility. With one of these systems impaired, a person may or may not be able to compensate for the missing component. If multiple systems are impaired, driving safety becomes an even greater concern. In particular, dementia and other cognitive impairments can seriously impair the brain's ability to integrate all the necessary information and react appropriately with split-second decisions.

Each state has a motor vehicle department that grants the privilege to drive to responsible and capable individuals. These departments can also revoke the license of anyone deemed unfit to drive. Laws about retesting as an individual gets older vary from state to state, but most states do not have mandatory retesting at particular ages. Therefore, older individuals can continue to drive, even when their driving ability becomes impaired, for as long as they hold a license. They may not be aware that one or more of their body systems is no longer functioning at an adequate level for safe driving. Every year, there are more motor vehicle accidents involving aging drivers who, it was determined in retrospect, should have no longer been driving.

Doctors in all states are required by law to report anyone with a physical or mental health condition that might impair driving ability. The state may then require the individual to get further evaluation and, if deemed necessary, will revoke the person's driving license. Many states will issue a "license" that looks similar but is for identification only. Many family members are actually relieved when a doctor reports their loved one's declining health to the state, because it spares the family from the task, allowing them to say it was out of their hands.

Driving and the independence it brings people are highly valued in American society, so when an individual's license is revoked, it can be a devastating blow that can precipitate depression.

Caregiver Burden

People with a chronic medical condition are often not the only ones experiencing the effects of the illness. Those who help out with caring for their needs, whether a spouse, other family member, or friend, can become exhausted, frustrated, and depressed from the caregiver burden. Caregiving spouses may also be suffering from their own medical problems, as well as having age-related limitations on their own stamina and ability to perform caregiving tasks.

Caregivers' burdens can be lightened when they are considered to be participating members of the health care team along with the medical doctors, psychiatrists, physiotherapists, nurses, social workers, and others. Ideally, caregivers should understand the illness and treatment options and be asked for input about various care options so that the best course of treatment is chosen for all parties involved. Caregivers also need to take care of themselves, both physically and emotionally. We give suggestions about care for the caregiver in chapters 3 and 4.

■ ■ ■

If You Are Concerned about Coping with a Chronic Illness or Disability

- Talk to a family member or friend.
- Learn as much as you can about your illness or disability.
- Follow your doctor's advice about regular follow-up visits, medications, physical therapy, and dietary and exercise regimens.
- Join a support group for the particular illness or disability.
- Socialize with other people who share similar interests.
- Maintain as much of your former lifestyle as you can, within reason. If you cannot do certain things, consider taking up new activities or hobbies that you are still capable of.
- Consider working with a psychotherapist. Approaches like problem-solving therapy (PST) have been shown to decrease the risk of becoming seriously depressed in the face of increasing medical burden because they help you learn better ways to cope and to understand your particular limits.

Suggestions for Family Members and Caregivers

- If, as a spouse, you are concerned about your loved one's mental outlook, reluctance to follow treatment instructions, driving safety, or any other issue, you can make an appointment for yourself to consult with your spouse's doctor. In most states, you need written permission from an individual to have a discussion with her doctor, but anyone can make a "one-way call" to warn a doctor about safety issues or risky behavior. The doctor takes the information under advisement to decide what, if anything, to do about it.

- If you are the caregiver, go along to appointments, ask questions, and take notes to remind yourself of the details later. Request specific permission to call on behalf of the person should something change in the meantime.

- Caregiving for a loved one can be hard work, and the stress of caregiving can also lead to anxiety, depression, or substance abuse. Be honest with yourself, and if you are feeling the stress, consider getting some extra support or help for yourself before serious depression results. Remember, your ability to give care depends on your own health, both physical and mental.

FIVE

Getting Relief from Physical Pain

The long and the short of chronic pain is how distressing it can be. Coping with and compensating for it requires energy, determination, and mental resources of exhausting proportions.

Many older adults experience persistent or chronic pain, since many conditions that cause pain—arthritis, cancer, heart disease—become more common with age; however, pain is not simply a consequence of getting older. On the contrary, it results from disability, injury, or illness, and therefore it can and should be treated. Too many older people think nothing more can be done or that they must simply be stoic when, in fact, a range of treatment options exist to alleviate or at least reduce their pain. In addition, dementia and other cognitive impairments can complicate the situation, making it more difficult for doctors and family members to adequately identify and treat pain. According to the National Pain Foundation, as many as 75 percent of seniors in care facilities and 50 percent of older adults living independently are dealing with chronic pain.

Pain, whether from disability or illness, can cause depression, and one symptom of depression is also physical pain. The two can circle endlessly, with pain contributing to depressive symptoms, and the depression making the pain feel worse. Chronic pain can also cause other problems, like sleep disruption and anxiety, which may lead to depression. Adequate control of chronic pain can improve overall quality of life and help relieve associated depression and anxiety symptoms. From the other angle, successfully treating depression, regardless of the cause, can lessen the severity of pain perception.

In this chapter, we begin with a brief discussion of common causes and complications of pain for older adults and then describe pain-management options, including both drug and nondrug treatments.

Understanding Pain

Painful arthritis is the most common form of chronic pain experienced by older people, as we briefly discussed in chapter 4. Other types of pain include chest pain (angina), migraine headaches, bone pain from various disorders, cancer-related pain, and neuropathic pain due to nerve damage. Sometimes pain is restricted to a particular location in the body, such as the back or a particular joint, but in other cases, it can occur simultaneously at multiple sites, such as with diseases like lupus (another autoimmune disorder that may begin with one organ and then progress to include others), polymyalgia rheumatic (an inflammatory disorder that causes muscle pain, usually in the neck, shoulders, hips, and thighs), and fibromyalgia (a disorder that causes bodywide pain in joints, muscles, tendons, and other tissues). Some brain injuries, like a stroke in a part of the brain called the thalamus, can produce pain syndromes as well. Last, psychiatric disorders such as depression, somatization disorder (in which a person has unexplained physical symptoms), and certain psychoses (in which a person loses contact with reality) can feature the intense perception of pain without damaged tissue or another discernible cause.

Different people experience and describe pain in different ways, such as dull, piercing, exquisite, lancinating, persistent, diffuse, or intolerable. There are clear variations in individual ability to tolerate pain intensity as well. Patients with severe, intense pain sometimes contemplate suicide to escape the pain. It's not difficult to see how chronic pain can lead to feeling depressed or anxious.

Pain that doesn't subside at night or that disturbs sleep quality can be particularly depressing. The restorative aspects of a good night's sleep can help an individual cope with pain and other adversities, while disrupted sleep—particularly chronically disrupted sleep from intrusive chronic pain—can lead to or exacerbate depression. Patients with chronic pain describe awakening in the morning feeling demoralized by the prospect of having to endure yet another day of pain without the ability to find relief.

Complications of Chronic Pain
Depression and Anxiety

People who are unable to participate as they formerly did in social or athletic activities or travel may experience depression as a result, on top of the already distressing situation of being forced to continuously confront the chronic pain itself. In addition, chronic pain that limits an individual's level of activity can lead to anxiety about being unable to carry out tasks like housecleaning, shopping, or maintenance.

> Mary, age 74, had been widowed for more than 20 years. Despite being on her own, she traveled extensively and had visited six continents on various guided tours over the years. She suffered from rheumatoid arthritis that had been diagnosed in her early 20s, so she liked guided tours because she could pay porters to carry her bags. She also liked meeting new people on every tour.
>
> When Mary took to her bed complaining of unbearable pain in her wrists, fingers, and shoulders, her daughter took her to the doctor. Mary repeatedly stated that the pain was so severe that she just wanted to die. She denied having any suicidal thoughts but cried out in misery that she could not live this way.
>
> Mary had had bouts of mild to moderate depression previously with similar complaints about pain, but she had never had a depressive episode as bad as this one. Her doctor prescribed an antidepressant that boosts two brain chemical neurotransmitters known to be involved in pain and depression (seratonin and norepinephrine) and told her that the medication might take a few weeks to achieve a full effect. The doctor also gave her another medicine to help her sleep at night; this helped her feel a little better within a few days, since she had also been sleep deprived.
>
> After four weeks with a gradually increasing dose of antidepressant, Mary reported that she not only felt her depression lift but that her joints were not bothering her nearly as much. In fact, she said she was searching on the Internet for her next tour. None of her arthritis pain medications had been changed.

As in Mary's case, depression can magnify or exacerbate the intensity of pain perception, while the successful treatment of depression helps relieve perceived pain intensity. Many patients report a reduction in the intensity of their pain when they're successfully treated for depression, even though nothing changed with the underlying cause of their pain. The reason that treating depression can alleviate pain has to do with pain signals and the brain.

Pain signals travel from our joints and muscles through nerve fibers to the spinal cord and then to the brain, where they are processed and interpreted or perceived as pain. The brain also sends out nerve signals to the spinal cord to suppress or dampen the pain signals, so that we can focus on other things than a constant stream of "updates" about every sensation. As an example of this phenomenon, think of a time when you were so preoccupied with an activity that you didn't notice sustaining an injury until later. The brain was suppressing the pain signals.

To use an analogy, pain signals flow through the spinal cord toward the brain like water through a garden hose. The brain's suppressive signals are equivalent to turning the tap down low to diminish the flow of water. When a person is depressed, the brain's suppressive signals are weakened—the tap is turned on fully, and the water (pain signals) flows more freely—thus increasing the perception of pain intensity. Successful treatment of depression restores or rebalances the normally present suppressive signals so that fewer pain signals reach the brain.

Other Complications

Many people with chronic pain, especially in their lower limbs or back, reduce and sometimes even cease physical activity, which is understandable if weight-bearing activity is uncomfortable. However, physical activity releases chemicals called endorphins, which are the body's natural painkillers, so being physically active can in fact help reduce pain. Other factors linked with physical activity can also help manage pain. For example, maintaining flexibility can help prevent joints from becoming frozen, and improving muscle tone can help keep joints, particularly vertebrae, in proper alignment with each other, thereby reducing the pressure on spinal nerves that protrude between each vertebra.

Pain and decreased flexibility in leg and foot joints can also lead to an increased risk of falls, and with the higher likelihood of thinning bones with advancing age, the result is frequently a fractured hip. Depending on how frail the individual is, a fractured hip can be fatal, because healing is slow, surgery is often required to stabilize the hip joint, and the patient is confined to bed, where he is at greater risk of contracting an acquired infection such as pneumonia or blood clots from inactivity.

Treatment and Management

The management of chronic pain frequently requires a multidimensional approach that includes some combination of the following:

- pain medication
- lifestyle changes, including losing weight, exercising, and improving sleep
- physical therapy, occupational therapy, or electrical stimulators
- injections of steroids and local anesthetics into joint spaces
- adequate treatment of depression and anxiety
- surgical intervention to relieve pressure on impinged nerves
- therapeutic massage, acupuncture, biofeedback, hypnosis, meditation, or prayer
- psychotherapy to learn better coping strategies

Finding the best combination of treatment and management options can take time and may require some trial and error. Also, pain relief medications, like all medications, carry risks and side effects. Some people with chronic pain conclude that enduring a certain degree of pain is preferable to the side effects (such as feeling sedated or less mentally sharp). In these instances, attention then shifts to lifestyle adjustments to better accommodate and cope with the pain.

All primary care physicians have training in how to manage pain, but they will often refer more difficult pain-management cases to a specialist or a pain clinic, where a group of professionals, including doctors, physical therapists, and sometimes psychologists, work together to formulate an effective chronic pain–management strategy. The treatment of pain is becoming increasingly sophisticated with the development of innovative treatment strategies.

Recent research has shown that a "stepped care" approach is most effective for finding the right treatment or combination of treatments that work best to control pain in a given individual. For example, if you begin with a medication strategy that eventually proves to be insufficient, then adding physiotherapy or psychotherapy may be beneficial. Caregivers who live with someone in chronic pain also have an important role to play. Pain control strategies that include the caregiver tend to be more effective than treatments that work with the pain sufferer alone. Controlling chronic pain can be a difficult goal to reach. It requires a persistent approach and a willingness to try various pain control strategies and combinations.

Medications

The first line of treatment for painful musculoskeletal conditions, such as arthritis or back pain, generally involves analgesic (meaning "to inhibit pain") medications, some of which can be purchased over the counter. An effective way to manage chronic pain with medications is to stay one step ahead of the pain. In other words, instead of waiting for a medication's effect to wear off and the pain to return, a better strategy is to time the delivery of the next dose of the drug to maintain a steady concentration in the bloodstream. Thus, the individual's pain remains suppressed, allowing him to function as pain-free as possible throughout the day and night.

ASPIRIN AND NONSTEROIDAL ANTI-INFLAMMATORY DRUGS

Aspirin treats pain, reduces fever, and has anti-inflammatory properties. One downside of aspirin is its ability to cause bleeding; for example, people with stomach ulcers are at greater risk of bleeding while taking aspirin. Taking too much aspirin at a single time can also produce hearing loss.

Nonsteroidal anti-inflammatory drugs (NSAIDs) include drugs like naproxen (Aleve) and ibuprofen (Advil, Motrin), which are available over the counter, and their cousins, the cox-2 inhibitors such as Celebrex and Celexecob, which are available only by prescription. The over-the-counter NSAIDs are generally safe when used occasionally for headaches or muscle and joint aches. For daily use, however, NSAIDs need to be carefully chosen by a doctor to reduce the risk of adverse effects. People with gastrointestinal conditions like ulcers or acid reflux or with a history of cardiac disease, stroke, or kidney disease should be carefully evaluated by their physician before using NSAID drugs on a daily basis.

ACETAMINOPHEN

Acetaminophen (Tylenol) is another over-the-counter compound that can reduce pain and body temperature, but it is not an anti-inflammatory. Acetaminophen is relatively safe and effective for use with chronic pain, although it does have the possible side effect of liver injury when taken in high doses or in combination with alcohol.

STEROIDS

Steroids, such as prednisone, are potent anti-inflammatory medications often used to treat flare-ups of conditions like asthma, rheumatoid arthritis, and multiple sclerosis. To reduce swelling or inflammation, prednisone is sometimes given in a regimen of decreasing doses over the course of days to weeks. Taking steroids over the long term can create a host of complications, however, such as brittle bones, diabetes, cataract formation, obesity, and increased risk of infection. Therefore, steroid use must be carefully monitored by a physician.

NARCOTICS

Narcotic medications (also called opioids or opiates) are powerful pain relievers that can also potentially cause a state of euphoria, or a "high." Narcotics like morphine are typically given after surgery to combat pain for several days until tissues begin to heal, and the medication is then withdrawn as the pain subsides. Narcotics are at times prescribed for long-term use, especially for severe disabling arthritis or pain that is not responding to NSAIDs. Narcotic medications frequently cause constipation, so individuals using narcotics should increase their fluid intake and consider using a stool softener or laxative to compensate.

Many people describe feeling loopy, spacey, or sedated from narcotic medications. Older individuals are also at risk of delirium and confusion while taking narcotics. Depression is another complication from chronic use of these medications. Narcotic medications may also cause pain fibers to adapt to pain signals over time, so increasingly larger doses are then required to control pain adequately.

Abruptly stopping chronically used narcotic medications can cause withdrawal symptoms, such as nausea, profuse sweating, runny nose, abdominal pain, and a craving for more narcotics to seek relief from this highly uncomfortable state. For some people taking narcotics for long-term management of chronic pain, the line between taking the medication for pain management and craving the medication for other effects, such as euphoria or reduced anxiety, can become blurred. Even when narcotics are initially prescribed to treat pain, some people become addicted to the medication and become highly anxious at the prospect of no longer having it. They may even make desperate pleas to their doctor or at emergency rooms for another prescription. For this reason, many primary care physicians don't prescribe narcotics for chronic pain, instead referring the patient to a pain specialist.

Given the trade in illicit narcotics like heroin, drug enforcement agencies are understandably strict about how narcotic medications are prescribed; in the United States, the Drug Enforcement Administration requires a doctor to have a special licensure designation in order to prescribe them.

LOCAL ANESTHETICS

Local anesthetics can be injected directly to a specific site to provide pain relief, such as when a dentist uses novocaine before drilling into an ailing tooth. These drugs are also used to relieve the pain of nerves trapped in various compartments within the body. Sometimes steroid drugs are injected along with the local anesthetic. Some individuals can get relief from back pain for many months with a well-placed injection, while others experience only short-lived relief, and continual injections become impractical.

ANTIDEPRESSANTS

Antidepressant medications have been used successfully to help alleviate chronic pain. Some antidepressants owe their antipain properties to direct effects on pain perception in addition to any antidepressant or antianxiety effects they have. They help restore the normal ability of the brain to suppress the intensity of pain signals coming from the limbs through the spinal cord to the brain. Antidepressants are commonly used simultaneously with antipain medications.

Nondrug Strategies

Nondrug strategies that have been effective for some people include electrical stimulation, which involves tiny battery-powered electrodes applied to the skin or surgically implanted. The stimulators produce an electrical stimulus that confuses pain fibers, thereby reducing the perception of pain. Reducing muscle tension and anxiety can also diminish the perception of pain and is the basis of Lamaze classes taught in preparation for childbirth. Biofeedback is another possible pain reduction strategy that uses special equipment to amplify brain waves and convert them to an audible or visual signal, which allows an individual to "learn" how to manipulate pain signals and diminish them.

Lifestyle changes that have been effective in reducing pain for some people include losing weight to decrease the burden that gravity places on painful joints; exercising to strengthen supporting muscles and maintain proper alignment of joints; using proper posture and movement techniques, such as bending the knees to lift objects instead of bending at the waist; and learning to pace physical activities. Improving sleep quality can also help an individual meet the daily challenge of coping better with pain (and vice versa). Other strategies listed earlier, including massage, acupuncture, hypnosis, meditation, and prayer have all been used successfully by some people to help make their experience of chronic pain more tolerable.

The brain itself has the ability to produce small amounts of compounds similar to narcotics like morphine. The brain releases these naturally occurring, narcotic-like compounds, called endorphins, in certain circumstances. For example, people who enjoy long-distance running describe a feeling of elation, or a "runner's high," which is thought to be the result of endorphins being released. Moderate levels of exercise will also trigger the release of some endorphins. This release may also be involved in the improved pain tolerance that can come from activities like meditation, acupuncture, and biofeedback.

Preventing Pain from Becoming Chronic and Disabling

Some sources of musculoskeletal pain can be prevented or minimized, especially lower back pain, which is a common complaint among American adults. Here are a few tips to keep in mind:

- Be physically active and maintain a healthy weight. Include muscle-strengthening and stretching exercises along with aerobic activities. Take time to stretch and warm up properly before exercising.
- Think about your posture, especially if you have to stand or sit for long periods. When standing, wear appropriate footwear, and when sitting, use a chair in which you can position both feet flat on the floor with knees and hips at the same level. A pillow behind the lower back can provide support where the back curves. Change your position frequently.
- Lift heavy items using your thigh or quadricep muscles and keeping your abdominal muscles tight rather than bending at the waist. Hold the item close to your body.
- Minimize tasks that require repetitive motions.

■ ■ ■

If You Are Concerned about Coping with Chronic Pain

- Learn about treatment and management options so that you can help determine your best strategy.
- See your doctor. Don't become resigned to severe pain; there are options for most people to control pain, even if it can't be eliminated altogether.
- Use some of the nondrug strategies mentioned above to help control pain.
- Stay as physically active as possible, eat a healthy diet, and get adequate sleep.
- Join a support group to avoid becoming isolated.

Suggestions for Family Members and Caregivers

- Be aware that the undertreatment of chronic pain is common among older individuals, so if you suspect that your loved one is receiving inadequate pain control, suggest that he speak to his doctor or ask for a referral to a pain specialist.
- If your loved one lives in a care facility, be an advocate for him with doctors and staff to ensure he gets adequate treatment for chronic pain.

SIX

Understanding Sleep and Fatigue

Once in a while, everyone has difficulty sleeping at night or is excessively tired during the day. When either one becomes a chronic condition, however, something is not right. Sleep is a biological and psychological necessity; without adequate sleep, people become fatigued, have little energy, concentrate and perform tasks poorly, become confused, and are prone to falling asleep suddenly during the daytime. Recent reports indicate that 74 percent of American adults are continuously sleep deprived.

Chronic insomnia—difficulty falling asleep or staying asleep—can lead to depression and anxiety. Conversely, insomnia can be one of several symptoms of depression and anxiety disorders. Chronic insomnia has other health consequences, too, such as an increased risk of becoming overweight and then subsequently developing diabetes. Safety concerns include greater accident rates and falling asleep while driving.

Older adults tend to experience more sleep disturbances than younger adults, yet their need for good quality sleep is no less. As people age, their sleep patterns tend to change. Older adults typically take longer to fall asleep than they used to, sleep less deeply, and wake up more frequently during the night. Their sleep cycle may also change so that less of their sleep is in the most restful sleep stages. Recent research has shown that about 10 to 15 percent of older adults experience insomnia by itself, and 30 to 60 percent suffer from insomnia combined with a psychiatric problem.

Insomnia and excessive daytime sleepiness are not normal parts of aging. Fortunately, there are several ways to address them. In this chapter, we discuss insomnia in detail, because it is the sleep disorder both caused by and leading to depression. We also briefly describe some other sleep disorders that can leave older adults feeling poorly rested, which in itself can contribute to feelings of anxiety or depression.

Sleep Disorders

A sleep disorder happens when normal sleep patterns or sleep stages are disturbed. Normal sleep is divided into rapid eye movement (REM) sleep, during which dreams occur, and non-REM sleep, which has four progressive stages. In stage 1, an individual sleeps lightly and can be easily aroused, while in stage 4, an individual sleeps deeply and gets the most restful and restorative sleep. During stage 4 sleep, heart rate and breathing slow down and body temperature drops by a whole degree, as if the individual is in a mild form of hibernation.

The most common sleep disorders in older people are insomnia, sleep apnea, and restless legs syndrome, but other sleep disorders can also occur, as listed in table 6.1. Sleep disorders can sometimes be identified by interviewing the bed partner, who may notice pauses in

Table 6.1. Sleep Disorders

Sleep disorder	Description
Insomnia	Difficulty falling asleep or staying asleep
Sleep apnea	Breathing pauses repeatedly while asleep
Restless legs syndrome	Abnormal sensations in the legs that can interfere with sleep quality
REM sleep behavior disorder	Physically acting out dreams while asleep
Sleep paralysis	Being awake but unable to move
Bruxism	Grinding teeth while asleep
Hypersomnia	Sleeping for an excessively long time at night or having trouble staying awake during the day
Narcolepsy	Involuntarily falling asleep during the day, usually for a few seconds or minutes
Jet lag or shift work	Temporarily changing the body's circadian rhythm, or internal clock, by traveling quickly across multiple time zones or by doing shift work
Parasomnias	Sleepwalking, nightmares, or night terrors

breathing indicative of sleep apnea or regular leg jerks that could be from restless legs syndrome.

Insomnia
Recognizing Insomnia

People with insomnia usually have difficulty falling asleep at night, or they wake up early and can't go back to sleep. In the morning, they generally feel poorly rested and then feel fatigued or sleepy during the day. Concentrating on tasks can be difficult. They may also experience tension headaches, be irritable, or have symptoms of anxiety or depression.

The causes of insomnia are numerous. The most likely reasons for insomnia in older adults are

- physical health problems, such as chronic pain or breathing difficulties
- mental health problems, including anxiety and depression
- medications, including antidepressants and heart and blood pressure medications, as well as over-the-counter medications for pain, allergies, or colds, which often contain caffeine or other stimulants
- caffeine or nicotine, which are both stimulants
- alcohol, which is a sedative but prevents the most restful stages of deep sleep
- the need to urinate during the night: some men develop an enlarged prostate gland (noncancerous), which increases their need to urinate frequently; women often have urinary incontinence, including feeling a frequent urge to urinate, as a result of pregnancy and childbirth; and anyone taking water pills or diuretics often needs to rise at night to urinate
- the hot flashes and night sweats that women experience during menopause
- a change in activity level, such as getting less exercise or taking excessively long daytime naps

Complications of Insomnia

People with chronic insomnia are at greater risk of becoming overweight or obese, which we discuss in chapter 9. They are also more likely to develop diseases like high blood pressure, heart disease, and diabetes, and these diseases may be more severe. The immune system may not function as well, leading to greater susceptibility to infections. Mental health problems, particularly depression and anxiety disorders, and substance abuse are also more likely to develop.

Individual reaction time gets slower when we have had inadequate sleep, and combined with the natural slowing of reaction times with age, the chance of having an accident increases while driving or operating other machinery or appliances. In general, quality of life declines for people with persistent insomnia, because they feel fatigued and irritable.

Treatments for Insomnia

Many people who go to a doctor with a complaint about insomnia expect to receive a prescription for sleeping pills. Sleeping pills are helpful for occasional insomnia, but they can cause psychological dependence and possible memory lapses. Sleeping pills should only be taken when someone has at least eight hours to spend in bed. One of our patients took sleeping pills to sleep on a five-hour plane trip and "awoke" disoriented at his destination, not being able to recall walking off the plane. The side effects of sleeping pills include excessive drowsiness, inability to think clearly, agitation, and problems with balance that can lead to falling. These side effects can be more severe in older people. Parasomnias, such as sleepwalking, can also be caused by these medications and lead to unusual or dangerous behaviors. For example, another of our patients reported driving his car to the local convenience store in the middle of the night before "awakening."

A preferable way to treat insomnia is to take a behavioral approach, which helps people learn new sleep behaviors and how to make their environment more conducive for sleep. Behavior therapies have recently been developed to effectively treat insomnia and thus avoid the potential long-term consequences of sleep medications.

Following a series of "rules" about good sleep hygiene, listed below, works well for many people with insomnia, provided that they apply them consistently. These rules are also sound advice for anyone wanting to maintain their ability to sleep well and prevent insomnia.

- Develop a regular schedule for sleep times. Go to bed at the same time every night, and get up at the same time every morning.
- Avoid exercising in the evening. Exercise increases adrenaline, a hormone that is stimulating and that can interfere with sleep.
- Avoid drinking alcohol in the evening.
- Avoid drinking fluids after a certain time in the evening (for people who wake up at night needing to urinate).
- Avoid eating before going to bed, and especially don't eat a heavy meal.
- Limit caffeine consumption after midday or eliminate caffeine altogether. Caffeine is found in coffee, many teas, energy drinks, and some sodas, chocolates, and over-the-counter medications.
- Eliminate intrusive noises and light. Try using ear plugs or wearing an eye mask.
- Use the bed only for sleep and intimacy. Don't watch TV or read in bed.
- After lying awake for 30 minutes, get up, sit in a chair, and read something not too stimulating. Avoid bright light. Go back to bed when this activity makes you feel sleepy. Repeat, if necessary.

This list of rules works for many insomnia sufferers if the rules are applied consistently, but simply handing the list to an individual is rarely enough. A more comprehensive technique uses cognitive behavioral therapy (CBT) to guide a patient in following strict routines that, over time, have shown remarkable success in improving or limiting insomnia. As with the sleep hygiene rules, the routines established during CBT must be followed properly. For example, the sleep specialist might ask a person to shorten her time spent in bed by a precise number of minutes daily to increase her natural tendency to sleep. It can take several weeks for the routines learned during CBT to improve sleep quality.

A technique called brief behavioral treatment for insomnia takes less time than CBT to resolve insomnia and uses a workbook approach to educate individuals about sleep hygiene and have them carefully track the exact times they are in bed and are asleep. A trained nurse practitioner reinforces the necessity to stick to the prescription for exact bedtime and rise time that is tailored to the individual. At the same time, the individual records and monitors sleep-related factors, including the length of time asleep, the number and time of awakenings at night, and self-ratings of daytime sleepiness. These data are then used to prescribe further steps.

Some people continue to experience chronic insomnia, despite instituting good sleep routines and being screened for sleep apnea, restless legs syndrome, depression, and other psychiatric disorders. In these instances, sleep medications may be necessary; the individual should be under the care of a physician knowledgeable in sleep medicine.

Effective management of insomnia through the various methods we've outlined can help reduce or even eliminate the anxiety and depression that often accompany insomnia. Conversely, adequate treatment of the medical or psychiatric issues that cause sleep disturbances can also eliminate insomnia by restoring the normal balance of biological rhythms necessary for good overall health.

OVER-THE-COUNTER SLEEP PREPARATIONS AND HERBALS

As insomnia is a common problem facing many adults of all ages, various companies compete to sell potential sleep remedies. Some of these preparations contain herbs, like valerian root extract, and may be harmless. They may even have some calming effect. Others, however, such as kava, have been known to increase bleeding in those who are at risk of certain bleeding disorders. Many over-the-counter sleep aids contain antihistamines, which are sedating but can also lead to mental confusion in older adults. Melatonin, a hormone produced naturally by the body in the absence of light, is another ingredient in some sleep preparations. For some people, taking melatonin daily is sedating enough to induce sleep, but in other people it doesn't work. Although melatonin is sold over the counter in the United States, it requires a prescription in many other countries on the grounds that we don't yet know enough about its safety.

As we discussed in chapter 1, claims made about the effectiveness of over-the-counter preparations and herbals do not equate to scientific proof. In addition, herbals are not regulated by the FDA for quality or concentration of active ingredients. Consumers must be aware of these limitations when considering whether to use herbals and other over-the-counter sleep aids.

Sleep Apnea

John, a 66-year-old retired salesman, had been an active golfer throughout his life, and he had been looking forward to playing golf daily in retirement. Unfortunately, his chronic back pain kept worsening, and he was demoralized to hear his surgeon tell him that more surgeries were unlikely to help and that physical therapy and pain management were now his best options. It got to the point where his pain exhausted him after playing just three holes of golf. He stopped going to the golf course and instead spent his time watching golf tournaments on TV. He said he never felt rested and had little energy, yet his wife noticed that he dozed off frequently. She also noted that he seemed to snack all day while watching TV, and after she confronted him about drinking too much beer, he switched to drinking a whole pitcher of sweetened iced tea every day.

At his next doctor's visit, John learned that he had gained 40 pounds since retiring a year earlier. His doctor discussed pain-management options and suggested that he cut back on the junk food between meals. He also sent John for a blood test to check his thyroid and suggested adding an antidepressant medication to his other pain medications. The doctor said the antidepressant would help reduce his pain as well as help his depressed mood. John didn't think he was seriously depressed, just angry and demoralized about not being able to enjoy golf as he once did.

Four weeks later, John went to his doctor for a follow-up visit feeling no better; he had gained another three pounds, too. His wife came with him this time and mentioned to the doctor that she couldn't sleep at night because John snored so loudly. She explained that he had always snored, but now it was like sleeping in a bear's den. She had to poke him in the ribs repeatedly to get him to roll onto his side to quiet his snoring, and one time, as she lay awake at 3:00 a.m., she noticed that he seemed to pause in his breathing for such a long time that she wondered if he was ever going to take another breath. After what had to be a full minute, he gasped, making a huge noise as he pulled in another lungful of air.

After listening carefully, John's doctor told them that he suspected John may have sleep apnea syndrome. He scheduled a sleep evaluation. John spent a night in a sleep lab wired to various monitors, and in the morning, he and his wife were amazed to hear that he had stopped breathing for a minute or more 44 times during the night. The diagnosis was confirmed as sleep apnea, which, in retrospect, explained his day-time fatigue and depressive symptoms as well. The sleep medicine specialist recommended that John use a continuous positive airway pressure (CPAP) device at night to prevent his airway from closing due to the increased tissue pressure on it from his weight gain. He also advised John to work hard at losing the excess 43 pounds of weight, saying that the sleep apnea might well disappear and that he would no longer need the CPAP. John agreed to see a nutritionist and now felt motivated to make a plan to lose the weight.

Six months later, John had managed to lose 18 pounds and, with the CPAP, was feeling much more rested in the morning. He had even begun a walking program, which helped strengthen his back muscles to the point that he was now able to play nine holes of golf. At his most recent checkup, he told his doctor that he was determined to lose the entire 43 pounds.

Sleep apnea is a disorder where a sleeping person stops breathing for a time and then starts breathing again. The word apnea means "cease to breathe," from the Greek *a-*, meaning "not," and *pnea*, meaning "to breathe." The most common type of sleep apnea, called obstructive sleep apnea, occurs because of profound relaxation of the throat muscles that allows throat tissue to narrow the airway and block breathing. Breathing ceases until the oxygen level within the bloodstream gets low enough for the brain to signal the need to gasp for air. The gasp allows the person to take a full breath, but in the process, she is awakened to a lighter level of sleep. As she relaxes again, the throat closes and the cycle repeats. The cycle can go on all night long without the person being aware of it, since she never wakes to full consciousness.

By continually being awakened to a lighter stage of sleep, the individual is deprived of the deepest, most restorative stage and thus feels poorly rested the next day and easily falls asleep during the daytime. Bed partners often say that they notice pauses for as long as two minutes in their partner's breathing, followed by gasping. The signs and symptoms of sleep apnea are loud snoring; having a dry mouth, sore throat, or headache in the morning; having trouble staying asleep (insomnia); and being very sleepy during the day (hypersomnia).

Older adults are more likely to develop sleep apnea than younger adults, and men are more likely than women, although the risk seems to increase for women after menopause. Obesity is a risk factor for sleep apnea, although people of normal weight can also have the disorder. Other risk factors include having high blood pressure, drinking alcohol, using sedatives, and smoking.

Sleep apnea has serious health consequences, because the repeated cycles of declining oxygen within the blood can cause pulmonary hypertension (increased pressure in the arteries carrying blood from the heart to the lungs) and subsequent heart failure. People with sleep apnea may also have complications with certain medications and after surgeries with general anesthetic.

When sleep apnea is diagnosed, several options can be considered for solving the problem. Since excessive weight is often an exacerbating or causal factor, significant weight loss can vastly improve or eliminate the problem. Quitting smoking can also help. For some people, a dental appliance that pulls the bottom jaw forward a fraction of an inch relative to the upper jaw works well to keep the airway open. The most common treatment is the CPAP machine, which maintains enough air pressure to keep the airway open and allow normal sleep in all its stages. With a CPAP machine, the sleeper wears an airtight mask attached through tubing to a toaster-sized device. The sleeper breathes on her own, but the increased pressure created by the machine doesn't allow the airway restriction to occur, thus eliminating the apnea episodes. Some people can't tolerate sleeping with the device in place, however. Last, surgical removal of excess tissue at the back of the throat can benefit some people as well.

Restless Legs Syndrome

Restless legs syndrome (RLS) is a poorly understood condition of abnormal sensations that can interfere with sleep quality. People with RLS get uncomfortable feelings in their legs and feet and occasionally in their arms when they are lying down or sitting for long periods. The sensations have been described as creeping, crawling, aching, tingling, bubbling, and pulling. Individuals feel compelled to move their limbs, and by doing so, they get temporary relief. The symptoms are typically more common at night and can last for an hour or longer. RLS is more common with age, and people with RLS often find that it gets worse as they age. The cause of RLS remains a mystery, but a low level of iron in the blood is one possible factor.

There is no known cure for RLS, but various medications have been used to successfully treat it, particularly the dopamine-boosting drug pramipexol (Mirapex). Opiate narcotics, muscle relaxants, some drugs used for Parkinson disease and epilepsy, and certain sleeping pills are other possibilities. Relaxation techniques, exercise, and avoiding caffeine, alcohol, and tobacco may also help decrease the intensity of RLS symptoms.

REM Sleep Behavioral Disorder

This disorder becomes more common with age, probably because of the aging brain and a breakdown of the normal ability of the brain to suppress motor movements while dreaming, which happens in REM sleep. During normal REM sleep, the muscles are limp and the body remains still. In some people, however, the mechanism responsible for inhibiting movement fails and causes REM sleep behavioral disorder.

People with this disorder flail their limbs and may speak or shout out during REM sleep, as if they are acting out their dreams. They can feel exhausted in the morning, and bed partners often complain of being kicked or punched. REM sleep behavioral disorder may be linked to other neurological conditions, including Lewy body dementia and Parkinson disease. Fortunately, this sleep disorder can usually be remedied by a small dose of a benzodiazepine medication called clonazepam (Klonapin), taken at bedtime. It may also be a good idea to make the bedroom safer with floor padding or bed rails.

■ ■ ■

If You Are Concerned about Your Sleep

- Make a sleep schedule and follow it faithfully, seven days a week.
- Use your bed and bedroom only for sleep and sex.
- Add some form of relaxation to your bedtime routine. For

example, you might ask your partner for a back or neck massage, take a warm bath or shower, or do yoga.

- Make your bedroom conducive to sleep: dark, quiet or with white noise in the background, and a comfortable temperature (usually cooler than room temperature).
- If you're lying awake and can't fall asleep, get out of bed and do a calm activity, such as reading something unstimulating, until you feel sleepy and then return to bed.
- Avoid napping during the daytime, or if you must, keep naps short and early in the afternoon.
- Be physically active every day, but not right before bedtime.
- Avoid eating too much late in the evening.
- Cut back or eliminate caffeine, alcohol, and nicotine.
- Avoid the temptation to use alcohol as a sleep aid, because it can have negative consequences for sleep quality.
- Find out if any of the medications you take, including over-the-counter products, have sleep disorders as a possible side effect.
- If you commonly get up during the night to use the bathroom, use night-lights or leave the bathroom light on to guard against the risk of falling (remove tripping hazards as well).
- Go to your doctor if these suggestions aren't helping you, or if you have trouble sleeping more than three times per week, with excessive sleepiness the next day.

Suggestions for Family Members and Caregivers

- If you're the bed partner of someone experiencing sleep problems, go along to the initial doctor visit in case you can give any details that may help make the correct diagnosis.
- Encourage the person to eat healthily, exercise daily, and follow the rules of good sleep hygiene.

SEVEN

Coping with the Loss
of a Loved One

Everyone will lose a loved one at some time in life. Grieving for that person is not only natural but necessary for most people, as they adjust to the new reality of living without the person. The word *bereavement* means to be deprived or robbed of something important and impalpable, such as security, love, and a future with the deceased person. Typical feelings during normal grief and bereavement are ones of sadness and sorrow, and even guilt and hostility. Other symptoms of grief include being preoccupied with images of the deceased person; taking on the traits of the deceased person; being unable to continue with day-to-day activities like work, hobbies, or taking care of dependent children; and experiencing physical distress, such as feeling waves of unfamiliar visceral pain (pain felt in the gut), increased anxiety, and insomnia.

The period of acute bereavement differs from person to person, with about two-thirds of grieving individuals beginning to return to their previous tasks and interests two to six months after their loss. For the other one-third, however, grief symptoms don't lessen over time and may even intensify, become debilitating, and may lead to anxiety or depression. Grief and depression are not the same thing, but grief is a risk factor for depression, and high anxiety frequently accompanies the adjustment that the surviving person must make. In addition, if an individual has had bouts of depression in the past, bereavement can easily trigger another episode. It can also worsen chronic depression or anxiety.

In this chapter, we describe normal grief and the typical feelings, symptoms, and behaviors that a bereaved person may feel. We then discuss the situation of grief turning into depression or complications, and the ways in which professional help can enable the bereaved person to return to leading an active life.

What Is Normal Grief?

Grief is an active process that requires a time and a place for the bereaved person to feel and sort through his emotions. The emotional energy that had been invested in the deceased person must be reorganized. The survivor may need to acknowledge or accept things like the meaning attached to his loss, the manner in which the person died, the untimeliness of the person's death, or unresolved areas of conflict or dispute. All of these issues can complicate the grieving process, as can the personality traits of the bereaved person.

In the first few months after losing a loved one, survivors go through a phase of acute grief, in which their daily lives may be disrupted by intense sadness, crying, poor sleep, and sometimes preoccupation with memories of the deceased person. A few grievers have visual hallucinations of the deceased person during the acute phase, and these hallucinations are not abnormal. For example, some people describe seeing the image of their late spouse standing at the foot of the bed when they wake in the night. The grievers may wish they could ask the image a question for help in coping with life alone. These hallucinations represent an intense wish by grievers to reach out to their loved ones again. Even when a pet dies, especially an elderly person's pet, people sometimes report hearing their pet's footsteps, which also represents the grievers' intense wish to be reconnected with the pet and to reestablish the comfort the pet brought them.

Rituals and behaviors are an important part of the grieving process in cultures the world over, and they take many different forms, such as wearing black clothing; performing elaborate ceremonies to honor the deceased; having family and friends sit with the griever for days and nights, reminiscing about the deceased; or hiring professional wailers. Some people have urges to search for traces of their loved one or to re-experience some of the feelings they had when in the person's company by going to favorite places they had shared. These behaviors, which are referred to as pining, generally diminish over time. Memorializing the dead person, whether by planting a tree, erecting a monument, or donating to a charity, is another behavior that can help the bereaved person to honor or preserve the memory of the deceased.

Not infrequently, well-meaning physicians prescribe sleeping pills or antianxiety medications to help individuals cope with the pain of their loss. These medications may be necessary in some cases, but they often blunt grievers' alertness and awareness throughout important events such as the funeral or memorial service. The painful emotions then return at a later time, possibly after family and friends have returned home and can no longer offer as much support. We suggest that it is most helpful to fully experience the emotions of grief during the funeral, when loving support is most available.

After the acute phase of two to six months, the bereaved person generally finds a new rhythm, although it can take as long as one to two years to feel comfortable with the reality of the loss and to invest energy in new activities. Grief never leaves completely, but over time it gets a little easier and occupies a place away from center stage. Seventy percent of grieving individuals progress on their own to a point of integrated grief, in which they acknowledge and periodically focus on their continuing sad and painful emotions about their loved one, but they also realize that they still have a life to live. Even when bereaved people have successfully integrated their grief into their lives and have been able to return to work, care for others, or pursue long-held goals, they will likely still experience occasional periods of grieving. Typically, grief can resurface on anniversaries, such as on the deceased person's birthday or the anniversary of the death. As grievers move toward integrated grief, the intensity of painful or negative feelings declines, and the risk of bereavement-related depression and anxiety becomes much lower.

After losing a spouse, some older individuals are clear in their mind that they had their "marital time" and are no longer interested in a new relationship. They feel content to live out their life as a widow or widower. Many other people who lose their spouse eventually confront the issue of forming a new romantic relationship. When couples have discussed this possibility before one partner dies, the surviving partner usually has an easier time dealing with it. People who had not had such a discussion often feel guilty about being with a new partner and worry that they are being disrespectful to their late spouse. The issue of dating again is often worrisome as well for individuals who have not dated for decades. They may feel uncertain about the prospect of a sexual aspect to a new relationship; we discuss sexuality in chapter 10. Some people are also apprehensive about entering another relationship for fear that the new partner will become infirm and require them to take on the burden of caregiving, or that the new partner will die and return them to an acute state of grief. Forming new relationships, whether platonic or romantic, is healthy and normal, however.

The support of family and friends, and for some people, the role of religious faith in their lives, is a critical part of finding a way to accept a significant loss and resume living. Many support groups and organizations are also dedicated to helping people through the pain of grieving (see the resources in this book). Professional counseling can also help people work through their grief, and especially help them understand any negative emotions that they're feeling.

When Does Grief Become Depression?

For about 30 percent of grievers, the symptoms of grief don't diminish over time and may even get worse. These people can become debilitated by depression, anxiety, post-traumatic stress disorder, complicated grief, or some combination of these.

Geraldine was 68 when her husband, Tom, succumbed to cancer. Geraldine had met and married Tom when she was 22 and had just finished teacher training. She never worked as a teacher, opting instead to devote herself to raising her and Tom's four children, one of whom, Jacob, was born with Down syndrome. Jacob occupied a great deal of Geraldine's time, since very few special services were available to help with his needs. Jacob also had an immune deficiency that made him prone to repeated infections.

Tom was a commercial airline pilot, so Geraldine was frequently home by herself with the children; however, Geraldine had grown up on a dairy farm and was no stranger to working long hours. She prided herself in continuing to run an organized household. She was also a devout Christian and remained active in her church, which she felt brought her strength to help all four of her children develop their particular talents to the fullest.

Tom and Geraldine had encouraged Jacob to be as independent as possible. As an adult, he was able to work at some custodial tasks, but he continued to live at home, since he couldn't drive, manage money, or problem solve very well. Jacob was frequently ill with pneumonia and died suddenly after a particularly severe episode at age 42. It was a hard adjustment for the whole family and particularly for Geraldine, who had devoted so much energy to Jacob's development and welfare. Tom retired several years later, and he and Geraldine spent much of their time visiting their remaining children, who were all now married and had their own children and lived in separate cities.

When Tom was diagnosed with cancer, Geraldine was certainly upset, but she quickly took on her familiar role of caregiver and diligently saw to it that Tom lacked nothing for his support and comfort. Tom slowly deteriorated over a three-year period and was bedbound for his last year. Geraldine refused Tom's doctor's offer to begin hospice care, because she felt that it was her duty and privilege to attend to her husband's personal care. She also had strong faith that his doctor would pull him through. As the months passed, Geraldine lovingly cared for her husband at home, even as he continued to weaken and lose weight. His doctor was no longer treating the cancer actively but providing palliative care to ease his pain. The doctor wasn't sure that Geraldine had "heard him," however, when he explained that Tom was dying.

When Tom died, Geraldine became distraught with grief and subsequently became severely depressed. Being so focused on Tom's care to restore him to life, Geraldine had not allowed herself to consider that he could die. Her grief persisted, but her three children, living elsewhere and busy with their own lives, didn't realize the toll their father's death was taking on their mother. Nearly a year after Tom's death, one of Geraldine's friends finally managed to persuade her to seek treatment. She eventually accepted an offer of psychotherapy to help her sort through and process her feelings. It became clear that she was dealing not just with her husband's death but with Jacob's death as well. Her preoccupation of 42 years with Jacob's care, followed by Tom's illness, had left little time for Geraldine to reflect or explore her feelings. She realized she was actually grieving for both of them, which intensified her bereavement.

It is not uncommon for people sustaining multiple losses to be overwhelmed by grief or to have a subsequent loss reactivate a prior one as the familiar feelings of grief return.

Grieving and depression can have similar features, such as feelings of sadness, disinterest toward usual activities, and impaired sleep or concentration. These symptoms are common in the acute phase of grief, especially during the first two months, so doctors generally avoid making a diagnosis of depression at this stage, even though some depressive symptoms are present. Even in these first few months, however, treatment of symptoms that qualify for a diagnosis of major depression may be appropriate if the griever has excessive guilt, slowed thinking or moving (psychomotor agitation), or any thoughts of wishing to be dead. If after several months individuals still find it difficult to function in daily activities, then they should seek professional help.

It is also not normal six months after losing a loved one for someone to

- be unable to focus on anything except the person's death
- be unable to accept the reality of the loss
- have grieving thoughts and feelings regularly intrude when trying to accomplish a task
- blame himself for the death or feel guilty about being alive
- feel like joy and happiness are impossible without the dead person
- feel like grief for the deceased person is all that is left of the person to hold on to
- feel depressed and unmotivated to work or socialize for weeks on end
- harbor any thoughts of wishing for death or thoughts about suicide

Having some of these features suggests that the individual may have complicated grief.

Grief and grieving are highly personal and varied experiences, but some scenarios do increase the chance of grievers becoming depressed and struggling with complicated grief as a result of their loss. For example, when a person dies as a result of an accident or a natural disaster, the survivors can experience intense shock. The death of a child is especially traumatic for parents, even when the child was already an adult. Suicide commonly causes feelings of guilt, and murder invariably sees the survivors searching for justice, which can complicate the grieving process.

Individuals with mental illness or mental disabilities may show an exacerbation of their symptoms when confronted with grief and often require additional mental health visits or adjustments in their medication to help them cope. People with Alzheimer disease or another dementia may have a distorted response to being told of a loved one's death, because they have trouble processing the news. Nevertheless, most people would agree that despite their cognitive impairment, people with mental illness or dementia have a right to know of the person's death. Finally, when an individual is dependent on another person for day-to-day needs and that person passes away, the dependent individual is at considerable risk of depression and panicky anxiety, especially if alternate plans had not been made for the individual's care.

Treatment for Bereavement-Related Depression and Anxiety

Research has clearly shown that bereavement-related major depression responds to treatment with antidepressant or antianxiety medications, which can help relieve some of the symptoms of grief that overlap with depression, such as sleep disturbance, loss of appetite, and poor concentration. The short-term use of sleeping medications is sometimes necessary but should be avoided long term by encouraging good sleep hygiene (see chapter 6). Other nondrug strategies to help restore a griever's overall function include reestablishing a regular rising time and bedtime to stabilize biological rhythms, reestablishing social connections, and avoiding self-medication with alcohol or other drugs.

Although helpful in many instances, medications do not help grieving individuals to grasp the meaning of their loss, and this is where psychotherapy can help. Psychotherapy allows grievers an opportunity to work through the emotions of grief, and many times, talking therapy is the only treatment needed. In other instances, a combination of psychotherapy and medication works best.

More specialized treatment may be required for people whose grieving is so intense that they struggle to cope with the reality of their loss and for people who experience intense anxiety mixed with depressive symptoms. About 10 percent of grievers become "stuck" in their grief, with no further progression or resolution of their symptoms. In all of these cases, individuals may benefit from a new form of psychotherapy called complicated grief therapy.

Complicated grief therapy involves helping grievers access thoughts and feelings about the person's death that are walled off because they are so painful to confront. Through specialized techniques and exercises, individuals learn how to better manage their grief while simultaneously reintroducing pleasurable activities and new goals. People experiencing complicated grief have also shown quicker and more complete improvement of their symptoms when complicated grief therapy is used in combination with antidepressant medications.

■ ■ ■

If You Are Concerned about Your Ability to Handle Your Grief

- Be proactive. Married couples can do themselves a great service by having a frank discussion about the reality of one partner passing away before the other. The surviving spouse can benefit significantly when a discussion has already taken place about where wills and other important documents are stored, the adequacy of and access to finances, living arrangements, burial and funeral preferences, and even the possibility of seeking new romantic attachments. Documenting advance directives can relieve the potential guilt feelings of making a wrong treatment choice in their loved one's last days. (We focus more on this issue in chapter 11.)
- Take advantage of your support network by speaking with family members, friends, or clergy.
- Stay physically healthy. Eat a nutritionally balanced diet, get physical exercise, and get adequate sleep and rest. Follow the guidelines for good sleep hygiene outlined in chapter 6.
- Avoid becoming isolated. Reestablish social connections. Participate in social activities. Join a support group. Some communities have support groups for specific losses, such as loss of a child or loss of a spouse.
- Avoid the temptation to self-medicate with alcohol or drugs.

- Plan ahead for anniversaries that might make your grief resurface.
- Consider seeking spiritual support from a place of worship.
- Go to a grief counselor. Your doctor may be able to recommend someone. Other places to look are the yellow pages, the Internet, a local grief support group, or a nearby branch of a professional society, such as the American Psychiatric Association or the American Psychological Association.
- See your doctor if you are having trouble coping and be open to trying antidepressant medication if it is prescribed.
- If you are a caregiver for a terminally ill loved one, consider seeking help with your anticipatory grief before the person passes away.

Suggestions for Family Members and Caregivers

- Invite the grieving person out for social activities.
- Offer to help with daily tasks like cooking, cleaning, and shopping.
- Suggest that the person see a doctor if the grief symptoms don't seem to be fading over time.
- Be content to just sit with the person at times; your mere presence may be comforting.
- Be willing to talk about how everyone misses the deceased person, especially at family gatherings or holidays, which are perfect times for remembrances and for offering support. Some families make the mistake of thinking that it will be too upsetting for the surviving widow or widower to talk about the deceased person when, in fact, the opposite is usually true.

EIGHT

Stopping Overuse of Alcohol or Prescription Drugs

For centuries people have used mind-altering substances to seek euphoria or to relieve pain. Used moderately, some substances—wine, for example—may even benefit health. When overused or misused, however, severe health problems, both physical and mental, result. Alcohol is the substance that most older individuals overuse, but prescription drug and tobacco addictions also cause serious problems. Some people drink more as they age because their daily lives have transitioned abruptly from one of active, scheduled, daily work to one of unscheduled retirement. Some feel bored, lonely, or socially isolated, or they may find themselves in more social settings with alcohol available. Retirement can dramatically increase the amount of time a couple spends with each other, and as a result, conflicts can intensify and lead to alcohol consumption as an escape.

Other individuals confronting declining mobility, chronic pain, physical illness, depression, anxiety, or grief may turn to alcohol or prescription drugs as self-medication. This situation can easily lead to addiction—the compelling need to continue using a substance despite recognizing the potential risks or harmful consequences. In other cases, individuals who have struggled for much of their lives with addiction may lose interest in drugs or alcohol as they become frightened by health or social consequences they can no longer ignore.

The physical health risks of excessive drinking—greater chances of heart disease, liver failure, and some cancers, among other risks—are better known than the long-term mental health risks. The overuse of alcohol or prescription drugs, however, can lead to increasing anxiety or depression when people become aware of the serious consequences yet feel powerless to control their substance use. Alcohol and drugs also contribute directly to a decline in brain function, with the combination of cognitive impairment and alcohol or prescription drug abuse leading to impaired driving, an increased risk of accidents and falling, outright confusion, disinhibition, and attacks of rage. Alcohol and drug problems in later life are often underdiagnosed and undertreated, yet treatment is available and can be of immense benefit to individuals and families.

In this chapter, we discuss the complications from overuse of alcohol, prescription drugs, and tobacco as well as available treatment options. We realize that the people most likely to read this chapter are not those with an addiction but rather family members or friends struggling with or concerned about someone else and wanting to know how to steer them toward help.

Alcohol Overuse

Everyone has heard news stories about possible health benefits from drinking moderate amounts of alcohol, which many studies do indeed support. For example, drinking a moderate amount of red wine every day can benefit heart health, and drinking a moderate amount of alcohol also seems to reduce the risk of Alzheimer disease, although the reason is unclear. The important point about potential health benefits, however, is that the consumption must be moderate, which the 2010 Dietary Guidelines for Americans defines as one drink per day for women and two drinks per day for men, regardless of weight, with "a drink" defined as follows:

- beer (5% alcohol): 12 fluid ounces
- wine (12% alcohol): 5 fluid ounces
- spirits (40% alcohol): 1.5 fluid ounces

Drinking more than a moderate amount of alcohol changes a person's consumption from use to abuse (see below) and, in some instances, to alcoholism. Surveys among the general population indicate that up to 15 percent of American adults age 50 and older are problem drinkers. In addition, in a recent 20-year follow-up study, 27 percent of women and 48 percent of men ages 75 to 85 exceed the recommended guidelines for alcohol consumption.

About two-thirds of older people with alcoholism began drinking at a young age. This group has more health consequences from drinking and is less amenable to receiving help than the other one-third, who began excess drinking later in life. The latter group often advanced to heavy alcohol consumption from social drinking or because of bereavement or another stress. They are more likely to accept intervention.

As people age, their bodies' ability to metabolize, or break down, alcohol decreases. Therefore, the amount of alcohol they used to drink can now have greater effects, including slurred speech, instability walking, poor quality sleep, and declining brain function. Gender makes a difference, too; older women who drink heavily are more likely to rapidly progress to alcohol-related illness than men.

Recognizing Alcohol Overuse

Dennis was 63 years old and drank heavily. He had started drinking regularly at the age of 14 and became seriously addicted to alcohol. He could see no reason for attempting to stop, even when his life began to fall apart years later.

He had married in his early 30s, and he and his wife had one son, Joshua. Although they were married for many years, his continual drinking became even heavier in his mid-50s, and his wife finally became fed up and divorced him. He subsequently lost his job and was forced into retirement. Now he lived alone in an apartment on his meager social security check. He didn't go out much and spent most of his day drinking. Joshua visited him regularly and tried to encourage him to cut down his drinking, but to no avail.

Dennis's health declined, and he developed a condition called cerebellar degeneration, in which chronic heavy alcohol use damages the brain and spinal cord and results in severe problems with balance and coordination. One day, Joshua came for a visit and found Dennis on the floor, where he had apparently been lying for perhaps a day or more. He hadn't been able to get up or get to a phone to call for help, and he was now quite confused from dehydration.

Despite medical treatment in a hospital, Dennis could no longer walk effectively and therefore could no longer live alone. Joshua found a place in a nursing facility and moved his father in. For the first time since age 14, Dennis was denied access to alcohol. After Dennis went through a successful detoxification treatment, Joshua—for the first time in his life—saw his father's real personality. Beneath a veneer of bravado and fierce independence emerged a much kinder, quite sociable individual, who was happy to help the nursing staff with small tasks. Dennis's forced sobriety allowed Joshua finally to get to know his father's real personality.

Someone who is unable to cut down or stop drinking, even when it is clearly causing health problems or disrupting family or work life, has an alcohol addiction, commonly called alcoholism. People with alcoholism have a compelling need to continue drinking despite recognizing the potential risks or harm. Their body has become dependent on the alcohol. The symptoms of alcoholism include

- feeling a strong need to drink
- being unable to limit the number of drinks consumed at one time
- drinking alone
- stashing alcohol in a desk drawer, car, or other unusual location
- needing to drink greater amounts of alcohol in order to feel an effect from it
- experiencing withdrawal symptoms (e.g., nausea, shaking) when alcohol is unavailable
- having blackouts, with loss of memory, when drinking heavily

It's also possible to have a drinking problem without having all the symptoms of alcoholism. In these cases, the problem is called alcohol use disorder and is defined as consuming more than the moderate amount of alcohol defined above. People with alcohol use disorder may have some of the symptoms of alcoholism, although they usually don't feel the urgent compulsion to drink or the withdrawal symptoms. Their bodies are not dependent on alcohol as they would be with alcoholism, but even so, people who abuse alcohol may still need help to quit drinking.

The American Geriatric Society recommends the CAGE questionnaire, developed by the Bowles Center for Alcohol Studies, to determine if a person abuses alcohol. The questionnaire has four questions:

1. Have you ever had trouble trying to Cut down your drinking?
2. Have you ever been Annoyed by other people's comments about your drinking?

3. Do you ever feel Guilty about your drinking?
4. Do you ever need an "Eye opener" drink to get going in the morning?

Answering *yes* to any of these questions indicates a significant alcohol problem.

Complications of Alcohol Overuse

Alcohol depresses the central nervous system, so it acts like a brake on the brain, slowing down its processes, including speech, coordination, balance, judgment, and inhibitions. With chronic heavy use, the body and brain become accustomed to the alcohol such that its immediate withdrawal can produce symptoms of intense anxiety or agitation, sweating, insomnia, and even visual hallucinations and seizures. Because of its slowing effect on the central nervous system, chronic alcohol overuse can contribute to depression. A recent study of people age 55 and older who had been hospitalized for depression showed that 37 percent also met the criteria for a diagnosis of alcoholism.

In older individuals in particular, alcoholism can lead to alcoholic dementia, with declines in cognitive function, especially memory, perception (visual hallucinations), and motor coordination (staggering when drunk, but also impaired nerve and spinal cord function). For people with signs of probable early Alzheimer disease or with symptoms of executive dysfunction (see chapter 3), the addition of alcohol can exacerbate or magnify any tendency to be impulsive, be quick tempered, show poor judgment, or use inappropriate social behavior.

Chronic alcoholism can also lead to various physical problems, including

- hepatitis and cirrhosis of the liver, and pancreatitis
- insomnia and lack of restorative sleep
- increased risk of infection
- high blood pressure
- increased risk of heart attacks, heart failure, abnormal heartbeat, and stroke
- osteoporosis (bone thinning) and increased risk of bone fractures
- vitamin deficiency, particularly thiamine (vitamin B1)

■ increased risk of some cancers (mouth, throat, liver, colon, breast)

Alcohol is a source of energy—many people are surprised by how many calories an alcoholic drink contains—so people who drink regularly often don't feel as hungry as they otherwise would. They eat less and can thus become nutritionally deficient. People with chronic alcoholism commonly have a vitamin B1 (thiamine) deficiency, which contributes to abnormal memory, impaired perception, and confusion.

Everyone is aware of the effects of alcohol on motor coordination, hand-eye coordination, and judgment that make driving after drinking heavily unsafe. The effect of alcohol on driving safety becomes even more pronounced with age, since people's reaction times naturally slow down as they get older. Older individuals are also more likely to have other problems, such as arthritis, undetected small strokes, or limitations in vision or hearing, which can make driving more difficult, even without alcohol.

People who take prescribed benzodiazepines (such as lorazepam, brand name Ativan) for anxiety have twice as many motor vehicle accidents as the general population and even more when they consume alcohol while taking this medication. Many medications carry warnings of toxicity when mixed with alcohol, and given that many older people take multiple medications every day, it is imperative to check with a pharmacist or physician about the risks of a particular mix of medications in combination with alcohol. Clearly, the safest option for anyone who plans to drive, regardless of age, is not to drink any alcohol.

Treatment for Alcohol Overuse

Many people who have alcohol use disorder or alcoholism do not recognize their problem. In these cases, family members or friends need to intervene to try to persuade a person to seek help. Sometimes a coordinated intervention is the most effective, whereby family members, friends, or coworkers each take a turn confronting the person with the drinking problem to give their impression of how the drinking has had a direct, negative effect on them personally. This type of multipronged confrontation is often more successful than individual confrontations, because it overwhelms the alcohol-addicted person's strong tendency toward self-denial. At the same time, the assembled group of people can offer the necessary support to get help.

For someone with chronic alcoholism, treatment first aims to remove the body's dependence on alcohol. Detoxification involves gradual withdrawal from alcohol using declining doses of sedative medications, all the while watching carefully for signs of withdrawal and treating them accordingly. Both inpatient and outpatient treatment facilities can provide the detoxification treatment, which typically takes three to seven days. Once individuals are successfully withdrawn from alcohol, counseling begins to address the issues in their personal lives that might have contributed to the addiction, such as marital discord, unhappiness with career choice, depression, or anxiety.

The most effective organization for helping individuals get control over their alcohol addiction and remain sober for the long term is Alcoholics Anonymous (AA). Another organization, Al-Anon, provides support for families and loved ones of people with alcoholism. Most communities have a chapter of AA (check the phone book or the website listed in the resources) as well as other drug and alcohol facilities where you can seek evaluation and help. Some facilities have special programs for older people, although most have one program to accommodate all ages. AA meetings offer support from counselors and other people with drinking problems who are maintaining sobriety. For people newly recovering from alcoholism, we highly recommend attending meetings daily in the first 90 days of recovery. Relapses are common, unfortunately, and sustained recovery often requires more than one round of rehabilitation.

Depression frequently coexists with alcohol addiction, either as a factor that led to the addiction or as a consequence of the addiction as it began to affect a person's relationships and job. Some drug and alcohol treatment facilities have dual diagnosis capabilities, where addicted individuals can receive simultaneous treatment for depression and their addiction. Adequate treatment of the depression is essential for achieving stable recovery, since relapse rates are higher among people with a dual diagnosis. Relapses are best prevented with group counseling that focuses on a thorough review of past substance abuse and its consequences, the triggers for drinking, and skills train-

Table 8.1. Medications Sometimes Used to Treat Alcoholism

Medication	Brand name	Action	Major side effects
Naltrexone	ReVia	Blocks receptors in the brain to alter the brain's reward system, which may be abnormally active in some people with alcoholism	Anxiety, appetite loss, chills, constipation, diarrhea, dizziness, drowsiness, headache, irritability, joint and muscle pain, nausea, sleeplessness, vomiting
Acamprosate	Campral	Reduces the craving for alcohol in some people, but the mechanism is uncertain	Diarrhea, dizziness, gas, loss of appetite, nausea, trouble sleeping, weakness
Disulfiram	Antabuse	Blocks a step in alcohol metabolism and causes severe nausea when alcohol is ingested	Drowsiness, headache, metallic or garlic taste in mouth

Source: Mayo Clinic Staff, Alcoholism: Treatments and Drugs (2010), www .mayoclinic.com/health/alcoholism/DS00340/DSECTION=treatments-and-drugs.

ing to deal with problems in ways other than by drinking. Long-term follow-up is also important. Some medications, listed in table 8.1, are also available as an adjunct to counseling and support groups to help individuals remain sober.

Preventing a Return to Alcohol Overuse

Alcoholism is an illness that can only be prevented by remaining sober. People who have successfully recovered from alcoholism should avoid alcohol altogether. Even one drink can be enough to precipitate a return to alcohol dependence. People can use many lifestyle strategies to remain sober. Those who are aware of drinking more than a moderate amount of alcohol can also make changes to their lifestyle to help them cut back on their drinking.

- Tell family and friends that you are not drinking so that they can be supportive.
- Participate in Alcoholics Anonymous or similar organizations.
- Change some of the social activities you participate in. Find activities that don't involve alcohol.
- At weddings and other unavoidable social gatherings where

other people are drinking, order a soda over ice with a twist of lemon or lime or a nonalcoholic beer, which has the malt beverage taste without the alcohol.

- Adopt a healthy lifestyle, including getting enough sleep, eating well, and exercising regularly.
- Consider learning yoga or meditation to manage stress.
- See a professional alcohol counselor for extra help.

Prescription Drugs

Prescription medicines clearly have their place in effectively relieving pain and acting on various ailments. Deliberate excessive use of these medications, however, is considered an addiction and often requires special treatment for both the addiction itself and any underlying condition, such as chronic pain, depression, or anxiety, that may have led to the drug abuse in the first place. Recent statistics show that prescription drug use exceeds marijuana use in people age 55 and older compared to those under age 45. Commonly abused prescription drugs are listed in table 8.2, along with their associated health risks.

People's use of prescription drugs often starts for entirely appropriate purposes, such as the treatment of pain, excessive anxiety, or attention-deficit disorder. If they then experiment with these prescribed drugs, they may find that the medications provide pleasurable effects, which become reinforcing. Prescription drugs that are sought out for recreation or to feed an addiction are often provided by unscrupulous pharmacists and physicians, as well as through theft and smuggling. Some people present themselves at hospital emergency rooms with various complaints, most commonly pain related, in an attempt to obtain more prescription medications to satisfy their addictions. Other people visit multiple doctors, who unknowingly each prescribe the medications that these "patients" are interested in.

Changes that commonly occur with aging affect the way the body metabolizes drugs. For example, the volume of blood and the amount of water in the blood decline, and the proportion of body fat increases. Thus, in aging individuals, a drug is dissolved in a smaller volume of fluid than it is in a younger person, making the drug concentration higher. Drugs that dissolve in fat accumulate in fat deposits, so the medication's effects are longer lasting, even after the drug

Table 8.2. Commonly Abused Prescription Medications and Their Health Risks

Medication type	Examples	Prescribed use	Health risks when abused
Sedatives and tranquilizers	Barbituates: Phenobarbitol; benzodiazepines lorazepam (Ativan), alprazolam (Xanax), diazepam (Valium)	Anxiety, sleep problems	Addiction, falls, mental confusion, accidents
Stimulants	Amphetamines: Adderall; methylphenidate: Ritalin	Attention-deficit hyperactivity disorder (ADHD), narcolepsy (a sleep disorder)	Anxiety, tremors, insomnia, seizures, paranoia
Opioid painkillers (narcotics)	Tylenol 3, oxycodone, morphine	Pain relief	Addiction, higher doses required over time for the same effect, severe constipation, sedation, mental confusion
Anabolic steroids	Various forms of testosterone and related compounds	Weight gain in the severely underweight, testosterone replacement for deficiency	High blood pressure, stroke, heart enlargement, liver toxicity, infertility, aggression, heart attack

Sources: National Institute on Drug Abuse, Prescription Drug Abuse Chart, www .nida.nih.gov/drugpages/prescripdrugschart.html, accessed June 24, 2011; Association Against Steroid Abuse, Dangers of Steroid Abuse, www.steroidabuse.com/ dangers-of-steroid-abuse.html, accessed June 24, 2011.

is stopped. Kidney and liver function also decline with age, which means that a drug can be toxic at a lower dose in an older person compared with a younger individual. Interactions between drugs also become more of an issue with older people, who are more likely to be taking multiple medications. Some of the health risks that can occur as a result of prescription drug abuse may, therefore, occur even with people who are taking their medications as prescribed, because of inadvertent toxic effects from drug interactions.

A common problem for people with memory deficits is the challenge of remembering to take their medications correctly. Forgetting to take a dose of medication leads to undertreatment, while "doubling up" (forgetting if the dose had already been taken and taking it again) can cause toxicity. Plastic medication boxes, available at any pharmacy, have compartments that can be filled for a week at a time with the help of a nurse or other family member, if necessary, and are an excellent way to ensure correct dosing and avoid forgetting doses.

Recognizing Prescription Drug Abuse

Recognizing dependence on prescription drugs can be difficult for family members or friends, especially when the person abusing the drugs has never had an addiction of any kind. Sometimes another medical problem develops and contributes to symptoms that then alert a family member or physician to the possibility. The case of Sandra illustrates how such a situation can develop, as well as the potential dangers of self-adjusting doses, mixing medications, and chronically using sedatives.

> Sandra was a 70-year-old retired insurance broker. She lived alone, having divorced 12 years earlier. She had dinner with her son, Jamie, and his family every month or so. Jamie described his mother as a hypochondriac. He knew that she was always ordering vitamin supplements by mail and had a medicine cabinet bursting with bottles of prescription drugs, accumulated over the years from various doctors she had seen. Jamie also knew that Sandra regularly sorted through the multitude of bottles and "mixed and matched" the contents to find the relief she was looking for. Nevertheless, Jamie wasn't particularly worried since his mother seemed to lead an active life, paid her bills on time, did her own yard work, and drove herself to visit other family members and friends without apparent problem.
>
> On Sandra's last dinner visit to Jamie's home, however, Jamie began to worry about her when she asked him for some Benadryl for her allergies; she said she'd taken her last two that morning. She also mentioned that her back was bothering her again, and to seek relief, she'd doubled her Tramadol pain reliever and had also taken a Valium pill left over from a time when she'd had muscle spasms. After hearing this list of pills that Sandra had taken during the day, Jamie advised against having a glass of wine with dinner. Reluctantly, she agreed.
>
> During the meal, Sandra didn't seem to be quite herself. She got mixed up when telling Jamie about what she'd been doing during the

week, and she referred to a mutual friend by the wrong name. Jamie was sufficiently concerned about her confusion that he insisted on driving her home later that evening. At 3:00 the next morning, he received a call from one of Sandra's neighbors saying that the ambulance was taking Sandra to the emergency room. Apparently, she had complained of being feverish and short of breath.

Jamie drove to the ER, where a doctor told him and Sandra that she had a small pneumonia, evident on her chest x-ray, and that he recommended admitting her for antibiotics and IV fluids. Sandra was admitted and seemed to be recovering, as her fever subsided and her alertness was improving, until three days later, when Jamie got another call. This time, the nurses told him that Sandra had suddenly become extremely agitated and wanted to leave in her hospital gown; they'd had to restrain her so she wouldn't hurt herself.

Jamie drove to the ER again, and on the way he stopped at Sandra's apartment and cleared out the contents of her medicine cabinet. He brought all 16 bottles to the hospital; 7 of them were sedatives, such as Valium, Xanax, and Ativan. With this new information, her physician concluded that Sandra's agitation was likely a symptom of withdrawal from abruptly stopping the chronic self-administration of sedating medications. He was then able to calm her with a sedative and begin a process of slowly tapering the sedative dose as a form of detoxification.

Some signs that prescription drug abuse might be occurring include an individual

- taking a higher dose than the doctor prescribed
- running out of medication early
- going to multiple doctors for the same complaint
- asking to borrow medications or stealing medications from others
- having difficulty sleeping or sleeping more than usual
- having slurred speech or other signs of confusion
- driving erratically, having accidents, or making errors in judgment
- being irritable or having mood swings
- displaying poor judgment

Complications of Prescription Drug Abuse

Different prescription drugs have different actions on the body when misused. Sedatives can produce alcohol-like disinhibition when taken in high enough quantities, as well as produce giddiness and a sense of well-being without anxiety. They can also induce severe sedation and sleep or even coma and respiratory arrest at higher doses, especially when mixed with alcohol. Like alcohol, these drugs can cause withdrawal symptoms of agitation, seizures, and even death when their chronic use is abruptly stopped.

Stimulants are mainly prescribed for attention-deficit hyperactivity disorder in children and adults. They are also used for combating the involuntary sleep episodes of narcolepsy and for people with residual daytime sleepiness caused by sleep apnea (see chapter 6). Stimulants are occasionally prescribed as an adjunct to depression treatment. Like cocaine, these drugs can produce a highly excitable state of body and mind, leading to a rapid heartbeat or an irregular heartbeat (arrhythmia), and their long-term use can sometimes induce paranoia or psychosis. Withdrawal from stimulant medications is not life threatening, but it usually makes the person feel rather depressed, sluggish, fatigued, and sleepy.

Narcotics (opioid painkillers) and their synthetic cousins have become the fastest growing category of abused prescription drugs. Morphine, isolated from poppy plants for over 200 years, is used as an analgesic for severe pain, but it also produces euphoria, which makes it attractive for drug abusers. Abuse of the synthetic narcotic oxycontin has risen to epidemic levels, as the pills are being sold by bogus "pain clinics" for profit. Narcotic painkillers are commonly used for postsurgical pain and as a last resort after trying milder remedies for severe chronic pain. The body quickly becomes tolerant of narcotics, however, such that higher doses are needed to achieve the same effect. The withdrawal from narcotic medications is intensely unpleasant, causing nausea, a runny nose, and severe abdominal pain, but it is rarely life threatening.

Driving while under the influence of a mind-altering substance is an obvious hazard, whether that substance is prescription drugs or alcohol, along with the increased risk for older drivers from physical limitations that can further impair driving ability. Doctors are required to report to the state licensing authority anyone whom they suspect has a mental or physical illness that would interfere with safe driving.

Treatment for Prescription Drug Abuse

Treatment for prescription drug abuse is similar to treatment for alcoholism in that the medications need to be slowly tapered, particularly in the case of sedatives, and sometimes the withdrawal symptoms need to be relieved with other medication for a period. The individual also needs to be evaluated and treated for conditions that may have led to the drug abuse, such as anxiety, depression, or early dementia.

For people who are so addicted that they're willing to do almost anything to obtain their drug of choice, the only option may be to try to limit their access by informing local pharmacies of the person's tendency to shop around to increase their supplies. Family members can also take the precaution of properly disposing of all legitimately prescribed drugs that are no longer needed, particularly unused narcotics, sedatives, and stimulants. These supplies can be a temptation for someone looking for drugs to experiment with or to support an addiction. Narcotics Anonymous (NA) and Nar-Anon are sister organizations to AA and Al-Anon and are designed to support recovery for drug abusers and family members.

Preventing Prescription Drug Abuse

When prescription drugs are used as prescribed, they don't commonly become abused. Unintentional drug abuse in older people can occur because of memory lapses or other problems, but people can minimize the chances of accidentally overdosing or becoming dependent on prescription drugs by

- following instructions for taking the medication
- using a pill box organizer to keep track of medications, especially when they take multiple medications at different times of the day
- asking for clarification about what the medication does and what to expect in terms of physical responses and side effects
- having medication doses double-checked by another person, for those with cognitive impairment

- telling their doctor if they have unusual or unexpected side effects
- disposing of unused medications by taking them back to their pharmacy or doctor

Nicotine: The Overlooked Addictive Drug

Nicotine occurs naturally in tobacco leaves and is another highly addictive drug. Individuals who enjoy smoking variously describe its calming and stimulating effects. It has become clear over the past several decades that inhaled particles, tar, and nicotine have serious effects on health, including increased risks of heart disease; stroke; lung, esophageal, stomach, and other cancers; and emphysema and other chronic lung diseases. Women who smoke have lower bone density after menopause. The risks of secondhand smoke have also led to public health laws prohibiting or restricting smoking in many public places.

Some people with chronic anxiety report that smoking helps them calm down, although its effect is short lived. According to one large study, people with more severe depression were more likely to smoke, and smokers with depression were less likely to quit than nondepressed smokers.

Kicking the habit of cigarette smoking is considered by many to be as difficult as stopping any other addiction. Strategies include alternative nicotine delivery systems, hypnosis, acupuncture, and recently, the prescription drug varenicline (Chantix). This drug blocks the craving for nicotine in some people, but it must be used with great caution (or avoided) in people who have suffered from depression, because it can induce or worsen depressive symptoms.

■ ■ ■

If You Are Concerned about Your Substance Use

- Tell a family member or friend.
- See your doctor.
- Call your local chapter of Alcoholics Anonymous or Narcotics Anonymous.

Suggestions for Family Members and Caregivers

- If you're concerned about someone's alcohol consumption, try talking to the person to find out how aware she is of her problem and whether she wants to seek help. If she does, support her in seeking treatment. Support can include offering to go along to appointments and inviting her to social occasions that don't include alcohol. If she doesn't recognize the problem, consider asking permission to make an appointment for yourself to see her doctor and discuss possible strategies that you could try. You could also try going to an Al-Anon meeting.
- For someone who denies that the amount of alcohol she drinks is a problem, try buying alcohol-free beer or offering to mix the drinks yourself and keep them light or even mix them with other strong flavors and eliminate alcohol altogether.
- For someone who may be taking too much medication because she forgets that she's already taken it, buy a pill box organizer and sort her prescription medications into it.

NINE

Maintaining Healthy Body Weight and Nutrition

Nutrition from food is one of the essential needs of the human body, yet for many people in today's society, the quantity and nutritional value of the food they eat is out of balance with their bodies' needs. Being overweight or obese—having excessive body fat—increases a person's risk of developing multiple diseases and other health problems. Obesity is now considered to be an epidemic in the United States. Data from the Centers for Disease Control and Prevention (CDC) indicate that in 2007–2008, one-third of adult Americans (20 years and older) were overweight, and an additional one-third were obese.

Depression and obesity are related to each other: being severely overweight can make a person feel depressed through dissatisfaction with body image or difficulty participating in activities, and conversely, being depressed can lead to gaining too much weight, usually by overeating to seek comfort. There may also be a hormonal link to the relationship, since the hormone cortisol is involved in the regulation of blood glucose and is often elevated with stresses like depression and anxiety. Feeling self-conscious about weight can also provoke anxiety, and some overanxious people use food to try to calm themselves.

Although there are many differing opinions about how the current epidemic of obesity has come about, it's clear that being overweight, and especially being obese, is physically and mentally unhealthy. Regular exercise, a moderate consumption of calories, and food choices that favor fresh vegetables and fruit can help control weight and improve mental health, physical health, and life expectancy. Those people who are able to achieve better control of their weight describe feeling more energetic, sleeping more restfully, and having greater self-esteem, exercise tolerance, social contacts, and libido (sexual drive).

The other end of the spectrum of unbalanced food consumption is malnutrition. Some older adults are at increased risk of malnutrition, which can in turn lead to problems with both physical and mental health. Malnutrition in older adults can be difficult to spot, but once recognized, it can usually be reversed fairly easily.

In this chapter, we first discuss symptoms, causes, complications, and treatment and management strategies for people who are overweight or obese. We then briefly discuss malnutrition and lifestyle habits that promote good nutrition and healthy body weight.

Recognizing Obesity

Charlotte was 67 when her doctor told her that she would soon need a knee replacement because of her osteoarthritis ("wear and tear" arthritis) if she didn't lose at least 30 pounds. Charlotte knew she carried excess weight, which she had slowly gained over the past 18 years, since her husband's death. She felt self-conscious and embarrassed about her weight and had purchased some pleated dresses to try to hide it, but they didn't seem to make much difference. She also noticed that her feet swelled more often than they used to, and she didn't sleep as well anymore.

Charlotte was the first to admit that she found comfort in food, frequently eating chips and ice cream to get through lonely evenings. Charlotte and her husband hadn't had children, so their social life had revolved around playing golf and spending time with friends who were couples. As a widow, Charlotte had declined to join the other couples they had known, so her circle of friends had shrunk. She had also lost interest in golf after her husband died, and now she did not exercise at all. Recently, she'd had to climb a hill to get to the cemetery at a friend's funeral, and she had been surprised to be completely out of breath, even though she didn't smoke.

Charlotte went to the medical clinic where she had gone for the past 30 years, and her doctor reviewed her records and plotted her weight on a computer. She pointed out a direct link between Charlotte's increased weight and the osteoarthritis in both her knees. Her left knee was the worst. This was when Charlotte's doctor warned her about the possible need for a knee replacement.

Charlotte was worried about her doctor's warning, and while talking it over with a friend, she realized she had not been taking care of her health. She needed to take responsibility since she had no one to rely on if she could no longer walk from arthritis. At her friend's suggestion, Charlotte joined a weight-loss group with the goal of losing 30 pounds. She liked and was inspired by the group's instructor, who had lost 52 pounds and had kept it off for 12 years. Charlotte learned to chart the food she ate using points and found out that she could still eat ice cream and potato chips, but they had to be counted in her weekly allowance of points.

After her first two weeks in the program, Charlotte was thrilled to have lost three pounds. For the first time since her husband had died, she felt a greater sense of control over her life. As well as learning how to count calories, read food labels, measure portion sizes, and plan for eating out, Charlotte was surprised by the wealth of ideas that she learned from other members of the group. For example, one woman mixed nonfat yogurt with artificial sweetener to make a tasty whipped cream substitute. Another woman mixed ricotta cheese with crushed pineapple and cocoa powder, froze the mixture in ice cube trays, and ate one cube each night for a low-calorie snack. Charlotte decided to combine these two ideas and stop buying ice cream.

She also came to understand that to lose weight, she had to burn more calories than she consumed, and that increasing her physical activity could hasten her weight loss. With her painful knees, she needed exercises that weren't hard on her knee joints. She tried water aerobics and the televised Sit and Be Fit classes, but then she joined her local YMCA and found that she really liked the spinning class on stationary bicycles. In one 45-minute period, she could see from the computer on the exercise bike that she had burned more than 500 calories. She took the spinning class three times a week, thereby burning 1,500 calories of extra fat.

As time passed, Charlotte had some weeks where she lost nothing or even gained a pound, which made her embarrassed to show up at the meetings. She was relieved to hear from other members that weight loss can sometimes follow that pattern. Nevertheless, by three months,

Charlotte had lost 15 pounds and was delighted to have achieved half her weight-loss goal. Charlotte told her friend that she had more energy, she was sleeping more soundly at night, and most important, she felt better about how she looked.

Body mass index, or BMI, is the most commonly used indicator of obesity. The formula is based on a person's weight and height. A BMI of 25 to 29.9 is defined as overweight, and a BMI of 30 or greater is defined as obese, as shown in table 9.1.

Genetic and hormonal factors, as well as drug side effects, can contribute to certain people having a higher than normal weight. Obesity usually results from a combination of several factors:

- poor eating habits, such as consuming a diet rich in high-calorie foods and beverages, eating large portions, and eating too quickly
- a sedentary lifestyle
- inadequate sleep, which can alter levels of hormones that regulate appetite
- older age, since hormonal and metabolic changes increase the risk of gaining weight, many people become less active as they age, and unless caloric intake also declines, they may gain weight
- some illnesses, such as a hormone disorder called Cushing syndrome, which can cause obesity as one of the symptoms; other conditions, like arthritis, can limit physical activity and thereby contribute to weight gain; mood disorders are well known to cause weight gain in some people (and weight loss in others)
- the side effects of certain medications, including some antidepressants, antipsychotics, and steroids
- social situation, since individuals are often influenced by the activities and weight of people in their social circle
- economic issues, which can include having such a limited income that it's difficult to buy healthier foods, or not knowing how to prepare foods in healthier ways

Of the factors in this list, the two greatest causes of obesity are consuming too many calories and not burning enough calories through physical activity. The excess calories become stored in the body as fat, which is an evolutionary adaptation of the human body to

Calculating Your Body Mass Index (BMI)

BMI = (weight in kilograms) / (height in meters)^2

or

BMI = (weight in pounds × 703) / (height in inches)^2

Table 9.1. Body Mass Index (BMI) Categories

BMI	Weight category
Less than 18.5	Underweight
18.5–24.9	Normal weight
25.0–29.9	Overweight
30.0 and greater	Obese
40.0 and greater	Extremely obese

be able to endure times of food scarcity. This situation was relevant for our ancestors but is less so for most Americans today, with our highly efficient food distribution system.

In addition to eating too many calories, we often ingest many calories from processed flour and corn sweeteners, in foods termed *hyperpalatable* by Dr. David Kessler, in his 2009 book, *The End of Overeating: Taking Control of the Insatiable North American Appetite.* Hyperpalatable foods tend to be combinations of fat, sugar, and salt. Generally, people eat more of these foods than they need, because they taste irresistibly good, and consume them very rapidly, not allowing enough time for the body's usual satiety or fullness sensors to trigger. The net result is that people regularly consume more fat and calories than needed to maintain their activity level.

Regular physical activity is low in American society in general, with many people relying entirely on their car rather than walking or using a bicycle, even for errands close to home. This problem is not limited to older people, but older individuals have a lot to lose from being too sedentary, including loss of bone density, flexibility, and joint health, as well as the overall negative effects of weight accumulation. Many American cities have been creating dedicated foot and bike paths to encourage people to exercise more and drive less.

Complications of Being Obese

Being overweight, and being obese in particular, substantially increases the risk of developing one or more of a long list of health problems, including

- abnormal cholesterol and triglycerides (a fat) in the blood
- type II diabetes
- high blood pressure
- heart disease
- stroke
- certain cancers, particularly colon, pancreas, and breast cancer
- poor circulation due to atherosclerosis (plaque deposits in arteries)
- osteoarthritis and gout (diseases that affect the joints)
- respiratory problems and sleep apnea (stopping breathing while asleep)
- fatty liver and cirrhosis of the liver
- depression

Obese people may also experience a lower quality of life if their weight restricts their ability to participate in activities. Physical disability, sexual problems, and social isolation can also be complications of obesity.

Metabolic Syndrome

In recent years, more and more people have been diagnosed with a set of features that together are called metabolic syndrome (and have also been called syndrome X and insulin resistance syndrome). Developing metabolic syndrome greatly increases a person's risk of diabetes, heart disease, and stroke. Someone with metabolic syndrome has at least three of the following metabolism disorders at the same time:

- Obesity, especially excess abdominal fat
- High blood pressure
- High levels of triglycerides and low levels of "good" cholesterol (high-density lipoprotein, or HDL)
- Resistance to insulin, which means that the body doesn't

respond normally to the hormone insulin, which helps regulate sugar in the blood

The risk of developing metabolic syndrome increases with age; people in their 60s have a 40 percent greater chance of being diagnosed with this syndrome. Other risk factors are race (people of Hispanic and Asian descent are at greater risk), obesity (a BMI over 25.0 increases the risk), a family history of diabetes, and the existence of other conditions like cardiovascular disease or polycystic ovary syndrome.

Treatments for Obesity

Although the prospect of trying to lose a significant amount of weight can be daunting, losing even a small amount can bring considerable health benefits and lower the risk of developing serious illness, such as metabolic syndrome. Losing as little as 5 percent of total body weight—10 pounds for a 200-pound individual—frequently allows a person to see and feel a difference in his health, which can then motivate a person to try losing more.

The primary methods for people to lose weight and then maintain a healthy weight are lifestyle changes, changing eating habits and behaviors associated with eating and increasing physical activity. For people who need additional help with losing weight and keeping it off, medications can sometimes be an option, and, rarely, surgery.

For people with metabolic syndrome, a combination of weight loss, a low-fat diet, more exercise, and medications to lower blood pressure, lower cholesterol, and improve glucose use by the body has been shown to delay or even prevent the development of diabetes. Individuals with metabolic syndrome should work closely with their personal physician to formulate a treatment plan and have progress monitored with successive blood tests.

Changing Eating Habits

Consuming too many calories and too many low-value calories tends to be a key problem for people carrying excess weight. The goal with changing eating habits, therefore, is to take in fewer calories and make those calories count toward better nutrition. (An individual who mainly consumes sugary drinks and carbohydrates like chips and cookies can actually be malnourished in terms of essential nutrients, despite taking in so many calories.)

It can be helpful to keep a record of everything eaten over a few days and then analyze where the calories are coming from. Easy culprits to reduce or eliminate in the diet are sugary beverages like sodas. Processed foods and foods with high sugar or fat content provide a lot of calories in a small quantity, making them dense foods. Fresh fruits and vegetables have fewer calories in the same quantity, so a person can eat more of them and feel fuller for longer without taking in more calories. Alcohol is another culprit that delivers a lot of calories quickly. Reducing alcohol intake can benefit other aspects of health as well as weight issues (see chapter 8).

Numerous quick-fix diets exist (just browse any bookstore shelf on weight loss), and many people have tried them with limited, temporary benefit or no success at all. Losing weight and then maintaining the lower weight cannot be achieved overnight or even over a few weeks. The most effective way to permanently and safely lose weight is to do it slowly: a pound or two per week is recommended as the safest rate.

With a BMI in the normal weight range and a sedentary lifestyle, women need an average of 1,500 calories per day to maintain their weight, and men need 1,800. To lose weight safely, women are recommended to consume 1,200 calories per day, and men, 1,500 calories per day. Normal BMI individuals need extra calories to maintain their weight if they are physically active, and for the same reason, weight loss will be hastened by doing extra physical activity without further decreases in caloric intake.

Changing Behaviors Associated with Eating

Losing weight gradually is as much about modifying behaviors as it is about reducing caloric intake. Behaviors associated with eating include how much we eat (large or small portions), how quickly we eat (fast or slowly), when we eat (a few large meals or smaller meals and more frequent snacks), and why we eat (for example, in response to anxiety or depression).

Portion size is crucial. Many dieticians and nutritionists recommend dividing the plate into two quarters and one half, with one quarter for protein, one quarter for carbohydrates, and one half for fruits and vegetables. Eating slowly allows brain receptors to receive the message that we are full or satiated, and we can then stop eating before taking in more food than needed. Eating small, healthy snacks between meals can help people manage their hunger and avoid eating too much at mealtime. Important with snacks, though, is to keep them small and low calorie, such as one piece of fruit, one cup of fresh vegetables, or two tablespoons of nuts or seeds.

If a person eats as a coping strategy for anxiety or depression, then knowing the triggers can help him understand when he is more likely to eat, with the goal being to learn how to substitute other ways of coping with the triggers. For example, if boredom during a long-distance drive is a trigger to stop at rest stops to eat high-calorie foods, then this behavior pattern might be broken by listening to an audio book to make the drive more interesting. Counseling, either individually or in a group, can help a person learn various coping strategies that don't involve eating. Support groups, such as Weight Watchers, can also provide motivation for people to work toward realistic weight loss goals along with other people in similar situations.

Increasing Physical Activity

Physical activity is the third key component of successfully losing weight and maintaining a healthy weight. When people first begin to lose weight, they usually have to start gradually and slowly increase the amount and type of physical activity that they do. There are many ways to begin being more active: walk instead of driving, get off the bus one stop earlier, take the stairs instead of the elevator, do some gardening or household chores.

The CDC recommends working up to 150 minutes (2½ hours) per week of moderate physical activity, such as brisk walking, water aerobics, or mowing the lawn. Several periods of 5 to 10 minutes of activity each day can add up quickly over a week and make the goal more achievable. Some people like to record their steps with an inexpensive pedometer and thus know whether they need to supplement their exercise regimen to meet their daily exercise goal.

The benefit of exercise is not limited to burning calories. For example, walking for just 30 minutes a day can drastically improve blood sugar levels for a person with metabolic syndrome, even if no actual weight loss takes place.

Medications

In some instances, medications may be advisable to help a person lose weight in conjunction with changing eating habits and behaviors as well as increasing exercise. Weight-loss medications aren't a substitute for making these lifestyle changes, however. The medications approved by the FDA work either by suppressing appetite or by blocking the absorption of fat in the digestive tract.

Surgery

Weight-loss surgery, or bariatric surgery, may also be an option in certain cases for morbid obesity, with a BMI greater than 50 and generally 100 or more pounds to lose. Again, it is not a substitute for lifestyle changes. For weight-loss surgery to be successful, the individual must be committed to changing eating habits and behaviors and increasing exercise. Surgeries include gastric bypass, gastric banding, and some other techniques, and they work by limiting the capacity of the stomach or decreasing the amount of food absorbed in the digestive tract. Weight-loss surgeries can cause significant complications and even death, so the decision to undergo this type of surgery must be made carefully and only as a last resort. Despite the stomach-shrinking effect of these procedures, 15 percent of individuals who undergo weight-loss surgery regain all their lost weight by eating smaller but more frequent meals.

Malnutrition in Older Adults

Some older adults develop health problems that increase their risk of becoming malnourished. For example, some chronic illnesses and medications suppress appetite or decrease the absorption of nutrients in the digestive system. People with dementia may no longer have the capability to determine how much or what types of food they need for adequate nutrition. Cognitive decline can also make it too difficult to do the multitasking involved in preparing meals, and many individuals with cognitive decline say they can no longer remember recipes, even for basic dishes that were their standards. Dental problems can also make it more difficult to chew or swallow.

Depression and alcoholism can both lead to diminished appetite, and alcohol's high caloric content often makes a person feel full but does not deliver nutrition (the archetypal "empty calories"). Older individuals often choose to eat the same foods habitually, thus reducing the variety that offers more complete nutrition. A restricted diet, such as a low-salt, low-fat, or low-sugar diet, can limit people's food options and make food taste bland. Some older adults also live on a limited income and may not be able to afford to buy sufficient food, while others lose interest in cooking or eating if they live alone.

Poor nutrition and vitamin deficiencies can lead to several other health problems, including

- fatigue and weakness, which can result in more falls and the possibility of bone fractures
- anemia, which is a low number of red blood cells and contributes to fatigue
- a weakened immune system, which increase the chances of contracting infections
- digestive system, lung, and heart problems
- impaired balance
- memory loss, depression, and even paranoia

Recognizing malnutrition can be difficult, especially since many older people naturally have a reduced appetite. Regularly spending mealtimes with an older person, however, can give family members an indication of whether they should be concerned. Physical problems that suggest potential malnutrition in individuals include bruising easily, having wounds that take a long time to heal, having problems with their teeth, and losing weight. Knowing what medications the person takes and whether they have side effects of reduced appetite or nutrient absorption can be helpful, too.

Family members can help improve an older person's nutrition by encouraging him to eat foods like nuts, nut butters, egg whites, cheese, fresh fruits, and fresh vegetables, all of which have high nutritional value. (Canned and frozen fruits and vegetables are second best, but they do lose some of their nutritional value during processing.) Making food taste more appealing may help, too, and can be accomplished fairly easily with herbs and spices. Salt may need to be restricted, however, for people with high blood pressure or congestive heart failure.

If social isolation is an issue, family members can invite their loved one over for meals and encourage him to join a lunch program or other group where people get together for a meal, such as those provided through many local seniors programs. Programs like Meals on Wheels may also be an option, where nutritious, prepared food is delivered regularly to the home for a modest cost. In the case of a tight budget, it may be helpful to suggest ideas for stretching money further while still buying nutritionally valuable foods. For example, buying bulk foods at lower cost and splitting them with someone else can save money. Last, family members can make an appointment to consult the person's doctor or dentist if they suspect that illness, medication, or other factors are contributing to their loved one's eating an inadequate diet.

Maintaining a Healthy Body Weight and Adequate Nutrition

A nutritionist or dietician can help determine an individual's ideal daily intake of calories and fat. Calculators are also available on several websites, which are listed in the resources section of this book. A nutritionally healthy diet consists of eating

- more fruits and vegetables, especially dark green, red, and orange vegetables
- more whole grains (e.g., 100% whole-grain cereal, bread, rice, and pasta)
- less meat, leaner meat, and only small portions of meat
- more fish and seafood (aim for twice a week)
- more beans and lentils, for fiber and protein
- less saturated fat (e.g., cookies, ice cream, cheese)
- less salt
- low-fat dairy products (which have as much calcium but less fat and fewer calories than higher fat products)

Some nutritionists recommend that people do most of their grocery shopping along the walls of the store instead of in the central aisles so that they buy more fresh foods and fewer processed ones.

Typically, fruits, vegetables, meat, seafood, and dairy products are along the walls, while processed foods are in the aisles. Also, it doesn't take much more time to check food labels, especially calories per portion, fat content, and salt content. The better options are those with fewer calories and lower fat and salt. Other strategies to get adequate nutrition while maintaining a healthy body weight include preparing your own food more often and eating out less often, sharing meals with family or friends, eating slowly, and drinking alcohol only in moderate amounts (a maximum of one drink per day for women and two drinks per day for men).

Although research studies favor eating a balanced diet with lots of fresh fruits and vegetables over consuming large doses of vitamin supplements, most health practitioners do suggest that people over age 60 take a multiple vitamin and mineral supplement daily to make sure they get the micronutrients that might be missing from their diet.

Being physically active conveys numerous health benefits, not just help in maintaining a healthy body weight. The CDC recommends that every week, older adults (defined as age 65 or older) without limiting health problems should do at least 150 minutes (2½ hours) of moderate aerobic activity, such as brisk walking, or 75 minutes (1¼ hours) of intense aerobic activity, such as jogging. In addition, at least twice a week, they should do strengthening activities for all major muscle groups. (Balance and muscle-strengthening activities also help lower the risk of falling.) Check with your doctor before embarking on a new exercise regimen to make sure it doesn't pose health or safety concerns.

■ ■ ■

If You Are Concerned about Your Weight

- Consider going to a doctor, nutritionist, or dietician, who can help you determine the right caloric intake for your body build and teach you strategies to lose weight.
- Keep track of what you eat and when you eat it. Writing it down can help you identify situations and times that trigger you to eat too much food or high-calorie foods so you can determine ways to avoid them.

- Keep track of your weight on a weekly basis (daily tracking is less effective, as weight fluctuates daily with water variations) to assess your progress. Weight and food intake records are valuable to review with a nutritionist to find out where you might be getting stuck. Regular reviews with a nutritionist can also help limit the demoralization from weight loss that is progressing slowly.
- Join a support group for weight loss.
- Ask family members and friends to support your efforts.
- Get into the habit of reading food labels and counting calories. Note that the calories listed on a package are often per serving, not per package.
- Commit to consuming seven servings of fruits and vegetables daily (preferably fresh for maximum nutrient value), as recommended by the FDA.
- Consider eating one vegetarian meal per week to reduce fat consumed from meat.
- Drink extra water, which helps promote a sense of fullness and helps with the metabolism of weight loss.
- Increase your daily exercise. Join a gym, pool, or other exercise facility. Many have programs aimed at older individuals, and some are women-only or men-only.
- Find a partner to exercise with you. The conversation helps decrease the tedium, and you can encourage each other to stick to a workable plan.
- Consider buying a pedometer to track the number of steps you take each day.
- If anxiety or depression are influencing how much you eat (whether too much or too little), seek effective mental health help to reduce or eliminate these triggers.
- Think long term and set realistic goals. Effective weight loss takes time.

Suggestions for Family Members and Caregivers

- Look at your own eating and exercising habits and make changes in support of the person you're concerned about.
- Consider making dietary changes together.
- Help the person find appropriate exercise options. Consider

making a commitment to support each other in doing more physical exercise together. For many people, walking is the easiest activity to begin with.

■ Encourage the person to stick to his lifestyle modification plans.

TEN

Preserving (or Renewing) Sexual Pleasure

As people get older, their sexual desires and abilities often change, but in no way does this mean that sex can no longer be a satisfying part of life. On the contrary, a healthy sex life, along with its physical and emotional benefits, can—and should, if it's wanted—continue as an individual ages. One survey of men and women between the ages of 60 and 91 showed that most of them (99%) expressed a desire for a sexual relationship, and 80 percent reported that they were currently sexually active. Some older people even report that their sex lives improve with age. Nevertheless, with aging, the intensity of sexual desire typically wanes somewhat, and sexual performance in both men and women can decline because of various medical and physical changes. The key to maintaining a mutually satisfying relationship is for partners to be open to talking about their needs and desires and to be willing to adapt to their changing physical abilities.

The relationship between sexuality and depression and anxiety can work in both directions. The physical changes within an aging body and mismatches in desire between partners can cause anxiety and are also potential risk factors for depression. On the other hand, depression and anxiety disorders can also interfere with normal sexual function.

In this chapter, we discuss the common medical problems that can affect normal sexual function as people age and some practical approaches for addressing them. We also suggest how family members or caregivers can deal with sexually inappropriate behavior in someone with dementia or other cognitive impairment.

Recognizing Obstacles to a Satisfying Sexuality

Sexual difficulties typically involve problems with desire, arousal, achieving orgasm, or pain associated with sexual intercourse. Although these problems can occur at any age, they more commonly occur in older individuals because of physical changes the body goes through with aging and the greater likelihood of older individuals having medical problems or taking medications that can interfere with sexual function. At any age, couples can experience sexual difficulties or frustrations because of differences in their sexual interests, such as the type or frequency of sexual contact. Understanding the reasons behind changes in sexual ability and interest can go far in helping people start a conversation with their partner or visit a doctor for treatment or advice.

Harriet and Sam enjoyed regular sexual intercourse throughout their married life and had been able to maintain their sexual activity despite Sam developing diabetes in his late 50s and suffering from partial erections, which were greatly helped by using sildenafil (Viagra). As Harriet passed through the stages of menopause in her late 40s, her sex drive was far weaker than it had been earlier in her life. Despite Harriet approaching 55 and Sam now in his late 60s and also feeling his sex drive waning, they still enjoyed sexual intercourse about once a month.

Sam saw an advertisement on television about "low T" (low testosterone) symptoms in men and how it lowered sex drive. On his next visit to his doctor, he asked to have his testosterone level checked, and it turned out to be below the normal range for someone in his age group. Sam's doctor reviewed his PSA (prostate specific antigen) test and reexamined his prostate gland to detect any possibility of cancer, and when these tests were normal, his doctor prescribed him little tubes of testosterone gel to rub on his chest after his morning shower, which penetrated his skin and increased the testosterone in his blood. Nothing seemed to happen for the first two weeks, but then Sam noticed that his sex drive (his libido) was becoming stronger. He was now approaching Harriet for sex as often as three times a week.

Harriet complained to one of her girlfriends that Sam's renewed vitality was causing her vaginal soreness and discomfort. She even confided that she almost wished Sam had never seen the "low T" advertise-ment. Harriet's friend replied that she was lucky Sam was still interested in sex, since her own husband seemed to be less so. Her friend sug-gested that Harriet visit her gynecologist in case there was something she could do to get rid of the discomfort in intercourse.

Harriet's gynecologist examined her and reassured her that her com-plaint was a common one. Being postmenopausal meant that she had less of the hormone estrogen circulating in her bloodstream than she used to, causing dryness in her genital area. Because Harriet had had a blood clot in her right leg (deep vein thrombosis) two years earlier, estrogen replacement pills were inadvisable, but her gynecologist reas-sured her that it was still safe for her to use a prescribed vaginal cream with a small amount of estrogen in it to help relieve the dryness. She also suggested that Harriet try a water-based lubricant during inter-course to increase her comfort. Last, her gynecologist suggested that Harriet let Sam know when sex was uncomfortable for her. Harriet said that she hated to limit his pleasure since he had struggled with weak erections since developing diabetes, but she agreed that they had al-ways maintained a good sex life by being respectful of each other, and that this new development was just one more thing for them to discuss and work through together.

Physical Illnesses

A period of illness can cause an unavoidable gap in sexual activity that may turn into a prolonged or even permanent drop-off, since couples are sometimes afraid to resume sexual activity. For example, after a heart attack, doctors caution against sexual activity for at least two months. After this recovery period, though, intercourse causes no more of a strain on the heart than walking up a flight of stairs. Lin-gering fears sometimes remain, however, and require patience and encouragement to resolve. The ideal first step is for the couple to speak with each other about their concerns and fears, either alone or with the guidance of a physician or counselor.

Other conditions can interfere with sexual performance or desire:

- High blood pressure, which can diminish the ability to become aroused

- Diabetes, which can cause erectile dysfunction (impotence) because of damaged nerves and narrowed arteries restricting blood flow to the penis
- Chronic pain, which can invade a person's life and eliminate all interest in sexual pleasure (see chapter 5 for more about dealing with chronic pain)
- Arthritis, which can limit movement and cause positional discomfort
- Hormone abnormalities, such as elevated prolactin levels, which can lower libido
- Impaired circulation in the blood supply to genital organs, which can limit the ability to achieve an erection
- Infections or cancer involving the sexual organs
- The need for an ostomy bag for bowel or bladder problems, which can make maintaining a workable sex life more challenging; similarly, any bowel or bladder incontinence raises anxiety about an accident during sex and prompts some people to avoid sexual contact altogether
- Obesity, which can make sexual intercourse more difficult
- Some surgeries, which can temporarily or permanently alter physical function; for example, some surgeries for prostate cancer can lead to permanent erectile dysfunction, and some gynecological surgeries remove the ability of a woman to have intercourse

Mental Illnesses

Depression and anxiety can contribute directly to sexual difficulty by decreasing or eliminating libido, or interest in sexual activity. The emotional energy required for a healthy sex life is often the first to be lost when someone becomes depressed. Anxiety disorders can also interfere with sexuality by causing or heightening trepidation about sexual performance. Conversely, a forced reduction in sexual activity, for any reason, can contribute to depression or anxiety, especially if it is accompanied by feelings of guilt or if it causes a mismatch in sexual desire between partners. Adequate treatment for depression and anxiety often has the effect of restoring libido, although it may be the last thing to return during the recovery process, after sleep, appetite, energy levels, and the ability to concentrate are restored.

Prescription Drugs

Many prescription drugs have the side effect of interfering with sexual function. In particular, the inability to achieve an orgasm for people who didn't have this problem before is usually due to medication side effects. Drugs that commonly affect sexual function (arousal, erectile function, or achieving orgasm) include

- antidepressants used to treat depression and anxiety disorders
- other psychiatric medications, such as antipsychotic drugs and lithium
- antihistamines for allergies, such as pseudoephedrine (Sudafed)
- high blood pressure medications and heart medications, such as digitalis (Digoxin)
- medications for treating the symptoms of Parkinson disease (although dopamine-increasing medications can sometimes increase libido, too)
- stomach acid blockers, such as the H2 blockers Tagamet, Zantac, and Pepcid
- some chemotherapy medications
- hormone medications, such as steroids, which can cause mood changes that affect sexual function
- hormone-blocking medications, such as those used in the treatment of breast and prostate cancers
- arthritis pain medications, such as ibuprofen (Motrin)
- opiate painkillers
- alcohol, nicotine, and other recreational drugs

If a prescription drug causes sexual difficulty as a side effect, it may be possible to reduce the dose, take a "vacation" from using the drug, or switch to another drug in order to preserve sexual function. None of these decisions should be made, however, without consulting the doctor who prescribed the medication. Consult with your pharmacist or physician to explore whether any medications you are taking might have potential sexual side effects.

A Woman's Aging Body

Menopause generally takes place between ages 35 and 55. During this process, the ovaries cease to produce eggs, and, more important, the production of the two sex hormones, estrogen and progesterone, declines to a very low level. The age-related decline in estrogen is associated with several physical changes that can affect the enjoyment of sex as well as the desire for sex. Most female readers of this book will likely have gone through the transition to menopause and be familiar with the common symptoms:

- hot flashes
- a pounding or racing heart
- insomnia
- mood swings
- declining sexual desire
- vaginal dryness
- increased abdominal fat
- loss of breast fullness

The declining estrogen level thins the genital tissues and reduces natural lubrication, so many menopausal and postmenopausal women experience some level of discomfort during intercourse that can be improved by using a topical estrogen cream applied to the genital tissues, as well as water-based lubricants during sexual intercourse. The emotional changes that accompany menopause can also affect a woman's interest in sexual activity, as can her concern about changes in her body shape or size.

A Man's Aging Body

The male sex hormone, testosterone (an androgen), controls a man's sex drive and performance. Testosterone, produced by the testicles, peaks in a man's late teens and early 20s and then begins to decline slowly. At about age 60, men typically begin to notice a waning of their sexual response. This so-called andropause, the male equivalent of menopause, can lead to decreased sexual desire and diminished erectile function, including the penis taking longer to become erect and the erection being less firm. A man may also take longer to reach orgasm. Erectile dysfunction (impotence), in which the penis cannot become erect or remain firm long enough for intercourse, becomes more common as men age. Other changes that men experience as a result of declining testosterone include reduced muscle mass, increased fatigue, and depression.

When One Partner Becomes the Caregiver

When someone has a physical illness, the person's partner may lose interest in sexual activity due to the stress of caregiving and the role change of becoming a caregiver. Talking frankly about the changes each partner is experiencing can help a couple adjust and adapt to their new reality. Setting aside the caregiving role from time to time to simply be the ill person's partner and allow for a mutually satisfying sexual encounter can be difficult to do, but with time and practice, doing so can allow both partners to fulfill their need for intimacy and perhaps even forget the illness for a time.

If one partner in a couple develops dementia and the other partner becomes the caregiver, sexuality can become problematic, especially as the illness progresses. When the caregiver remains cognitively normal and continues to have normal sexual desires, sexual activity can present a dilemma. Caregivers often become concerned about whether they are "taking advantage" of their partner, who may no longer be seen as a fully consenting partner because of cognitive impairment. Similarly, as a partner becomes more dysfunctional from dementia and is no longer available for sexual intimacy, caregivers may struggle with the desire to form romantic or sexual connections with other (cognitively intact) people.

Treatment of Sexual Difficulties

Going to a primary care physician is appropriate for questions or concerns about disorders of sexual desire or a decline in sexual function. This physician may be able to advise the individual or may make a referral to a gynecologist, urologist, endocrinologist, psychotherapist, or sex therapist.

For Women

Estrogen replacement therapy, or ERT, can minimize some of the changes that occur during menopause. Oral estrogen supplements and estrogen-containing cream applied to the genital area can relieve vaginal dryness and thinning tissues, making sexual intercourse less uncomfortable and more pleasurable. Over-the-counter vaginal lubricants used during intercourse can also help when vaginal dryness is an issue.

Oral ERT needs to be considered carefully since it can increase the risk of breast and uterine cancers, as well as the risk of forming blood clots. The decision about whether to use hormonal replacement should be an individual one made between a woman and her physician, after taking into account any other risk factors and fully understanding the risks versus the benefits.

Libido in women is driven by testosterone-like sex hormones, similar to those in men, which women naturally produce in low levels in the adrenal glands and which can decline with age. Thus, loss of libido in women can sometimes be improved by small amounts of testosterone replacement, sometimes given in combination with estrogen.

For Men

Low levels of testosterone can be boosted with testosterone replacement given orally, by injection, or in a patch or gel applied to the chest for absorption through the skin. There are potential risks with replacing testosterone, such as promoting further growth of prostate tumor cells in men with prostate cancer. Before considering testosterone replacement therapy, a man should be screened for prostate cancer with a blood test called prostate specific antigen, or PSA, as well as through a rectal examination of the prostate gland.

Although Viagra is the most commonly known medication to help men experiencing erectile dysfunction, several other medications are also available. The medications work by allowing increased blood flow to the penis during sexual stimulation.

These medications have been highly beneficial for many men, but they don't work in all cases. For men who are unable to achieve an erection with medication, another option is to consult a urologist about a device that creates negative pressure or a vacuum to help achieve an erection. As a last resort, a urologist can surgically implant a device that replaces the normal erectile mechanism with an artificial one.

Sex Therapy

When a medical evaluation reveals no physical abnormality, or when interpersonal difficulties are clearly related to an unsatisfying sex life, sex therapy may be the appropriate treatment. Sex therapists use various techniques to help couples rekindle their interest in sexuality by slowly building their sensual sharing. For example, a couple may be asked to spend quality time together giving each other backrubs but avoiding more direct sexual contact. As each partner's comfort improves, the level of intimacy then changes to include other behaviors, such as kissing, hugging, and fondling, but still without intercourse allowed. The goal of these step-wise exercises is to increase comfort gradually and allow a progression of natural excitement, so that sexual love making will take place in an atmosphere of mutual respect. Eventually, the couple progresses to include mutually satisfying intercourse in their sexual activities.

Being Sexual without Intercourse

Occasionally, intercourse is no longer possible for an individual. For example, irreversible impotence that doesn't respond to drugs like Viagra can be a complication of surgical removal of the prostate gland for treating cancer, and women who undergo certain types of gynecological surgery can no longer have intercourse. However, these situations don't necessitate an end to sexual activity. Instead, a person's definition of what constitutes sexual contact may simply need to be expanded.

Many people believe that sexual activity must culminate in intercourse, but other intimate activities such as hugging, kissing, fondling, and oral or manual stimulation can be sexually satisfying and can allow for orgasm without sexual intercourse. In fact, older adults who remain sexually active often report that although they engage in intercourse, they place a stronger emphasis on more subtle forms of intimacy. Some couples enjoy sharing erotic books, videos, or sex toys as enhancements to their sexual experience. Sexual contact without orgasm can also be mutually satisfying between partners who agree that the activity adds emotional closeness and pleasure to their relationship.

Self-stimulation, or masturbation, is normal and healthy at any age, and it may be the only sexual outlet if no partner is available. One study reported that in their 50s, 66 percent of men and 47 percent of women masturbate, and in their 70s, the figures are 43 percent of men and 33 percent of women.

Ultimately, couples who are able to adapt to their physical circumstances and are willing to try to expand their definition of mutually satisfying sexual contact can maintain an intimate connection and avoid a mismatch in sexual desire that may otherwise lead to distress, depression, or anxiety.

■ ■ ■

If You Are Concerned about Your Sex Life

- If you're in a relationship where a sexual difficulty has become evident, try talking with your partner about it. It may be easiest to start a conversation in a neutral place and fully clothed. Talk about your own feelings and thoughts, such as "I like it when you hug me," rather than framing your comments as being about the other person, such as "You don't hug me anymore."

- Consider changing your definition of sexual activity to explore other ways of sharing intimacy with your partner. You could consider including more touch (holding hands, kissing, cuddling, and stroking); different positions (get ideas from a book; if you are uncomfortable going to the library or a traditional bookstore for this type of book, try an online bookstore); or vibrators and lubricants.

- Talk to a doctor. Discussing sexual problems can be difficult and embarrassing for many people, but try to put these feelings aside. Your doctor is there to help, and you won't be the first patient with a sexual concern. The chances are good that your doctor can help you manage a medication or condition that is interfering with your sex life or can refer you to a therapist or other specialist who can help you deal with emotional or other issues affecting your sex life.

- If you're single and interested, consider seeking a partner. Older individuals may feel awkward, shy, or simply out of touch with dating and meeting people for potential romantic relationships, especially if they have recently lost their longtime spouse or have been single for many years. Nevertheless, the effort of socializing and participating in activities can be worthwhile when you do meet someone you connect with. When beginning an intimate relationship with a new partner, it's always important to practice safe sex, however; sexually transmitted infections don't discriminate by age.

Sexual Inappropriateness: Suggestions for Family Members and Caregivers

Aging individuals with cognitive impairment, particularly executive dysfunction (as discussed in chapter 3), often show signs of disinhibition. Their disinhibition can lead them to make insensitive remarks or jokes or to act in ways that other people regard as overly flirtatious, sexually aggressive, or otherwise inappropriately sexual for a particular social setting. The coexistence of cognitive impairment with hypomania or mania (the "up" phase of bipolar disorder), or with the additional disinhibiting effects of alcohol or other drugs, can further contribute to unwanted or inappropriate sexual commentary, groping behaviors, and other unwanted advances.

Strategies for family members to cope with this problem begin with learning about why the behaviors are occurring, as well as making matter-of-fact attempts to educate the person with dementia if she is able to comprehend. Limiting access to alcohol can reduce disinhibition. Behavioral strategies like intervening immediately when the unwanted behavior occurs, to put a stop to it, or disallowing the individual's access to certain people or situations might be required. As a last resort, some medications may be effective at reducing impulsivity, such as seratonin-boosting antidepressants like paroxetine (Paxil). In very rare and desperate instances, sex hormone manipulation can be tried to reduce sexual desire.

Sexually inappropriate behavior can also occur in care facilities, where people are sometimes sexually attracted to each other even if they are still married to a spouse who lives elsewhere. The effects of dementia can lead to misidentification, confusion, and just plain forgetting who they are attached to in marriage and what is and isn't socially acceptable. People in later stages of dementia live more in the moment. Family members can become understandably angry and bewildered when a loved one with dementia "pairs off" with another person in a care facility setting. Families need to understand that such behaviors happen because of their loved one's illness mixed with the universal human desire for attachment. Family members sometimes conclude that the comforting or satisfying aspects of these pairings offset any impropriety.

ELEVEN

Planning for Life's Final Phase

A source of anxiety for many people as they get older is how they will live out their final years, especially if they become seriously ill or disabled. Being prepared and letting people close to you know your wishes can remove much of the anxiety. In addition, having clear instructions about medical interventions and living arrangements can remove the guesswork for family members, allowing them to help you be treated in the way that you want.

In this chapter, we discuss advance directives, long-term care options, and making a last will and testament.

Advance Directives

Isabella, age 68, swore that she would not allow herself to "linger on" as her mother had. Her mother had been on life support for months after a severe stroke, and she never woke up. She was kept alive with liquid nutrition through a feeding tube and with a ventilator that breathed for her when she developed pneumonia. At the time, her mother's doctor wouldn't hear of "unplugging" her to let her die; he professed to hold hope that she would one day wake up. Isabella was distressed but had no recourse and could only watch helplessly until her mother finally died in her sleep one night from an apparent heart attack.

When Isabella discussed her wishes with her own physician, he directed her to a list of lawyers who specialized in advance directives. She went to a lawyer who recorded her wishes not to be resuscitated if she had a stroke or heart attack, not to be placed on a breathing machine, and not to be fed by a tube if she could no longer feed herself. Isabella wanted to be sure that her end-of-life wishes were carried out, and with no living relatives, she left copies of her advance directives with her doctor, lawyer, neighbor, and priest. She even carried a copy in her purse.

Nine years later, Isabella lost consciousness while shopping, and paramedics began life support measures after determining that her heart had stopped. They transported her to a nearby hospital emergency room, where personnel worked on her heart for an hour before it stabilized. Blood tests came back showing that Isabella had had a massive heart attack. Six days later, Isabella's personal physician heard what had happened and immediately called the hospital to tell them of Isabella's wishes and send them a copy of her advance directives. The hospital was uneasy about accepting the document, so Isabella's physician had her transferred to the hospital where he worked, and after he personally attested to the authenticity of her advance directives, Isabella's life support was stopped, and she was allowed to slip away as she had wished.

Advance directives are documents that record a person's preferences about medical treatment if he is unable to make decisions himself. Ideally, an advance directive describes how the individual wants to be treated in various situations, such as in the event of being permanently unconscious (in a coma). Today's sophisticated technology for life support can keep a person's heart beating and maintain breathing, but although these efforts can be truly life preserving in someone whose overall health is likely to recover substantially, this scenario isn't always the case. Many people would not want to be kept alive if their chances of recovery were extremely unlikely. In these instances, an advance directive can tell doctors and family members which treatments to withhold. Of course, an advance directive can also indicate which treatments a person does want to have. Advance directives are legally binding in most states, but it is important to check with a knowledgeable legal resource in your state, particularly if you have moved across state lines.

There are several types of advance directive: living wills, powers of attorney, and do-not-resuscitate orders.

Living Will

A living will, sometimes called a healthcare declaration or healthcare directive, indicates the medical treatments and life-saving interventions that a person wants to receive, as well as how long any

Table 11.1. Major Types of Lifesaving Interventions

Intervention	Description
Cardiac resuscitation	Restarts the heart when it stops beating and may include mouth-to-mouth breathing, chest compressions, electrical shocks, intravenous drugs, and other techniques
Pulmonary ventilation	Breathes for a person who no longer can; a machine inflates and deflates the lungs through a tube in the windpipe
Kidney dialysis	Removes toxins and wastes from the blood and excess fluid from the body using a machine
Nutrition and hydration support	Provides nutrients and fluids either intravenously or through a tube into the stomach

interventions should continue. Quality of life and what constitutes a minimum function to describe someone as "alive" is an ongoing ethical debate. Most people would agree that an individual with body functions but without brain function has no quality of life, and some hospitals mandate that such individuals be removed from life support and allowed to die. Sometimes, however, family members are unable to give up on a hoped-for recovery; there have been cases of individuals living for decades in a coma, with costly round-the-clock care. Nearly everyone, of any age, should complete advance directive documents, to specify what kind of care and interventions they want at the end of life. These forms are available free from the attorney general's office in every state. The major types of life-saving interventions are shown in table 11.1.

Medical Power of Attorney

A living will cannot designate another person to make medical decisions; for this, a separate legal document is required to appoint a medical power of attorney (POA), sometimes called a durable power of attorney. A medical POA is appointed by an individual to make medical decisions on his behalf should he become so ill that he's unable to make the decisions himself. Because a living will is unlikely to include all possible situations, it can be helpful to designate a medical POA in addition to having a living will. In this instance, the POA would follow the living will and make decisions only in circumstances not specified in the will. Some people don't write a living will and only appoint a medical POA.

Some appointees don't want to have sole responsibility as medical POA, preferring to share it (between two adult children, for example). Sharing POA responsibility for medical decision making means, however, that disagreements can arise, and in the worst cases, a deadlock can occur over granting permission for a particular intervention or procedure. Nonetheless, in our experience, concerned family members usually confer with each other and make joint decisions anyway, and the designated POA is then the person who communicates with the medical team.

When people have dementia and their ability to make sound decisions is in question, or they are deemed at risk of being the victim of fraud, the medical POA can take over decision making. Deciding the right moment to step in as POA, however, can be extremely difficult for family members, particularly when the person with dementia cannot recognize his lapsing judgment. Unfortunately, people with dementia sometimes makes accusations against the POA, saying, for example, that the POA is stealing their money or forcing them into a care facility.

A medical POA doesn't have to be a family member. People can designate anyone whom they trust to understand their wishes and advocate for them. Note that a medical POA is not the same as a financial POA, with legal authority to pay bills, access bank accounts, and perform other business transactions, unless the individual specifies the same person to act as POA in both ways.

Do-Not-Resuscitate Order

A do-not-resuscitate (DNR) order is a request for cardiopulmonary resuscitation (CPR) to be withheld if a person's heart stops beating or if he stops breathing. DNR orders are placed into a person's medical chart, either with his doctor or at the hospital where he's being treated. They are recognized in all states.

Making Sure Your Advance Directives Are Followed

Terminal illness and death aren't topics most people want to dwell on, but putting the necessary details on paper in a legal document makes your preferences clear and takes some of the burden off family

Guardianship and Power of Attorney Are Not the Same

The term *guardianship* is often confused with *power of attorney*, but the two are fundamentally different. Granting somebody guardianship of another person is a legal decision made by a judge in a court of law, transferring decision making for the individual in question to the designated guardian without requiring the individual's consent. Because guardianship takes away a person's right to self-determination—a basic right granted by the U.S. Constitution—the laws governing guardianship were designed to protect vulnerable people from exploitation. Guardianship is usually granted only if an individual is unable to care for himself and decisions need to be made to provide for his safety and welfare, such as medical treatment or placement in a care facility. Guardianship also allows the individual's financial resources to be made available to pay for any needed care.

Guardianship cases typically involve an older person with advanced dementia living on his own, without adequate community or family support, and deteriorating to the point where his behavior endangers his health. In rare cases, a severely ill person who was deemed to require guardianship later recovers adequate function to be independent again and seeks to rescind the guardianship. Most often, however, guardianship remains in place for the remainder of the individual's life.

Sometimes family members are forced to pursue guardianship for a relative who clearly cannot care for himself but refuses every reasonable offer of assistance. In such instances, the court considers the opinion of psychiatrists, statements from family members or neighbors, and a statement from the individual, if he is able to give one. These cases are rarely contested, although some are. The guardian need not be related to the individual. For example, in some states there are charitable or religious organizations whose mandate is to assist when no family members are available to take on the role of guardian, or when family members are unwilling to do so.

The preferable situation is for people to designate their power of attorney while of sound mind to avoid a future scenario where having a guardian appointed is determined to be necessary.

members at a difficult time. Discussing your advance directive with key family members ahead of time can help avoid any misunderstandings or surprises that could jeopardize your wishes being carried out.

Any document is only of use if it is available at the right time and in the right place. A copy of your advance directives should go to your primary care physician, spouse, family members or trusted friend, and lawyer. Having an accessible copy at home and taking one to the hospital if admitted are also good ideas.

Many people choose to have a lawyer draw up their advance directives. Lawyers who specialize in elder law can be found in yellow pages listings or through a local legal services office or bar association. Although a lawyer can ensure that an advance directive is written in language that won't be misinterpreted, it isn't necessary to use a lawyer. Each state has an advance directive form that can be filled out and signed in the presence of witnesses. Forms can be obtained from various organizations, like the National Hospice and Palliative Care Organization (listed in the resources section) and from local or state public health departments.

Another option is to use the Five Wishes document (see the resources for a website address), which meets legal requirements for an advance directive in 42 states; in the other eight states, a Five Wishes document can be attached to the state's required form. The document can be purchased for a nominal fee and is often provided by hospice agencies to their clients. In addition to information about health care decisions and medical treatments, the document includes information about what the individual wants his loved ones to know.

An advance directive can be revised or changed at any time by filling out the forms again, having the new directive witnessed, and asking anyone with copies to destroy the old one and replace it with the new one.

People who are in committed relationships that are not legally recognized should ensure that properly filled-out medical POA documents specifically authorizing a given individual to have decision-making power are in place well in advance of their potential need. Otherwise, given the current health care privacy laws, health care personnel may not recognize the rights of partners in these relationships to make decisions or sometimes even to gain entry to intensive care units or other treatment settings.

Long-Term Care Options

Long-term care includes a wide range of options, from day programs to round-the-clock nursing care. It can be a difficult prospect for anyone who values his independence to consider long-term care, but for many people and their families, some form of care assistance becomes necessary. The best situation is to learn about the options in advance and make inquiries and plans before you need the services. Doing so can help reduce anxiety and give people time to mentally adjust to the idea of accepting assistance for various activities, thus lessening the chances of becoming depressed at the time of the transition. People who are unaware of the options and financial considerations with long-term care can find themselves having to make a hasty decision if a sudden illness or injury occurs. In these cases, the chance of becoming anxious or depressed is much greater.

Long-term care options to consider:

- Home care providers, also called home health aides, who offer services like bathing, dressing, grocery shopping, meal preparation, and basic housekeeping. Some can also provide limited medical care. Home care providers may visit a person at home once or twice a week or daily, depending on the arrangements made.

- Day programs, which are ideal for people who don't need extensive care. They provide a social setting for older adults through group meals and activities. The services provided by day programs vary greatly, but some programs offer transportation, field trips, exercise classes, and limited medical assistance, like dispensing medications and taking blood pressure readings.

- Rental apartments designed for seniors. These buildings are built and maintained for ease of access and with safety issues in mind to lower the risk of residents falling. Some of them have wheelchair-accessible apartments with lowered sinks and countertops. Most senior apartment buildings have a common area for socializing, and some offer hot meals at low cost, housekeeping, and transportation services.

- Assisted living facilities, where residents typically have a private or shared room, and staff are available to assist them if necessary with needs such as taking medications, bathing, and dressing. Staff are on call to give assistance round-the-clock if a resident requires help, and many assisted living facilities have a registered nurse on staff. Assisted living facilities also provide meal and housekeeping services, as well as transportation, activities, and possibly amenities like barbers and hairdressers. There are also memory care assisted living facilities that specialize in assisting people with Alzheimer disease and other dementias that affect memory.

- Nursing home facilities, which provide 24-hour nursing care for people who need more assistance than provided by an assisted living facility. As well as providing meals and assistance with daily living activities like bathing and dressing, nursing home care includes assistance with certain medical needs, such as changing wound dressings and giving injections.

- Retirement communities, which are facilities that offer a range of services from senior housing through round-the-clock nursing care, often in different buildings but on the same campus. Residents of these facilities can move from one level of care to another as they need it. Living at a retirement community can be expensive, but for those who can afford it, this type of care can bring peace of mind by removing all decision-making burden from adult children.

Because there is such a range of options—and even the level of services provided within any one category can vary significantly—people should think about their likely needs and their preferences for facility size, living arrangements (private or shared rooms), services, and activities. In addition, facilities may have rules about things like visiting hours, which will be important to some people. The cost of the care facility is also a factor for most people; we discuss insurance and payment options later in this chapter.

Another consideration is the proximity of the facility to family and other support. The potential stress of moving into a care facility can be greatly eased by supportive family who can visit frequently to offer quality time beyond the basic care provided by the facility. Home cooking, outings, familiar companionship, and the ability to attend family functions or see grandchildren can make an enormous difference in residents' mood and acceptance of their new living arrangements. Family members can also provide an important advocacy role to negotiate with facility staff and administrators about medical care and other decisions. Of course, for some people, the increase in social contact and activities, the availability of helpful staff, and the diminished hardships of struggling with daily living come as a welcome relief.

When deciding whether a particular facility may be suitable for you or your loved one, make an appointment to tour the facility and look for cleanliness, how comfortable the furniture and rooms are, whether the residents seem happy, how the residents are treated by staff, and the staff-to-resident ratio. You may also want to make unscheduled visits.

If you are a family member looking into long-term care options for a loved one, try as much as possible to involve the individual in discussions and decisions. Doing so can ease the transition to the new arrangements, and after all, provided the person does not have advanced dementia, he continues to be a freethinking individual with preferences and concerns.

Financing Long-Term Care

Long-term care can be exceedingly expensive, especially for people who opt for in-home services. For example, somebody needing round-the-clock care would need three shifts of staff every 24 hours, so the cost could easily exceed $100,000 per year. Even someone needing assistance at home for only a few days per week could expect to pay several thousand dollars annually; from a recent survey, Genworth Financial reported that in 2011, the median rate across the United States for licensed home health aide services was $19 per hour. Day programs often charge a daily rate, with an average cost in 2009 of $67 per day, according to the U.S. Administration on Aging. Assisted living and nursing home facilities typically charge a monthly rate. Some facilities have an all-inclusive rate, while others charge extra for certain services or activities. For example, the U.S. Administration on Aging reports the 2009 average rate of $3,131 per month for a one-bedroom unit in an assisted living facility. Facilities with more amenities can cost twice as much.

If personal savings are insufficient to cover the costs of paying for long-term care, there are some other options. Long-term care insurance can help preserve assets and alleviate the fear of running out of money, as well as protect adult children from the financial responsibility of paying for their parents' care. Long-term care insurance is generally paid as monthly premiums and can be used to cover nursing home and other care services. Premiums and coverage vary according to a person's age, so premiums are lower when a policy is purchased by a younger person. For a person of advanced age or who has already become infirm, the cost may be prohibitively high, or a policy may not even be available.

Medicaid, a state and federal government program, assists people who have limited financial resources to pay for care. The services that Medicaid covers vary by state. Medicare, a federal government program, covers various medical costs for people older than 65 and for people with certain disabilities. Medicare may pay for limited nursing home care and certain home care services. The Older Americans Act is a federal government program that may pay for some long-term care as well.

Palliative and Hospice Care

Two other types of care are palliative care and hospice care. Palliative care provides services to help improve the quality of life for people with serious or terminal illness, when a cure is no longer possible or when active treatment of the underlying medical condition offers no chance for improvement or stabilization. A care specialist can help treat an individual's symptoms, particularly chronic pain, ease the side effects of treatment, and assist with emotional and other issues. Palliative care specialists also help family members get a better understanding of the illness, communicate with doctors and other health professionals, and assist the move from hospital back home or to a nursing home. Palliative care may be covered by private and long-term care insurers.

Hospice care focuses on providing comfort and support to both the terminally ill person and the family members in the final weeks or months of the ill person's life. Typically, treatment options have been exhausted for people receiving hospice care, and the care specialists aim to manage their pain and help with their physical, emotional, and spiritual needs. A lot of hospice care occurs in the home, with a care specialist visiting the person, but it can also be provided at hospitals, nursing homes, and hospice facilities. Hospice care also offers bereavement services and counseling to family members, both as they anticipate their loved one's passing and after he passes away. Medicare and private insurance may pay for hospice care, if a physician makes the referral and certifies that the individual has a terminal illness and six months or less to live.

Arranging Your Affairs in Advance

When a loved one dies, the remaining family members may encounter a distressing amount of paperwork. Finding all relevant documents, such as a last will and testament, insurance policies, property deeds, bank accounts, financial investments, safety deposit boxes, and sometimes even hidden valuables can be a daunting task. People who organize their records and have a list of account numbers and locations make the job so much easier for their family and help ensure that assets are transferred according to their wishes. Every year, in fact, millions of dollars in assets go unclaimed and sit in bank accounts long forgotten. Most people would undoubtedly prefer their family members to make use of these assets. A copy of bank account details and other information should be kept in an easy-to-find place, with a second copy left with a lawyer, trusted friend, or family member, or in a safe deposit box at a bank.

Last Will and Testament

To be confident that your assets and personal property are transferred as you wish, it's advisable to write a last will and testament—and not just older adults. All adults should have a will, even though as many as 60 percent of American adults don't have one, according to a recent survey by FindLaw.com, an online division of Thomson Reuters. A last will and testament is a document intended to state a person's wishes about distributing his property and assets after his death, as well as to give details about his wishes in terms of a funeral service, burial, and so on. If there is no will (or one cannot be found), the assets remaining after payment of debts and expenses are distributed according to "next of kin" rules established by the state the deceased lived in. Although some people don't see the need for a will, not having one can result in severe family tension and divisions over distributing assets, not to mention expensive legal battles.

A will generally names an executor to ensure that all outstanding bills are paid, inheritance taxes are paid, and remaining assets are distributed to the people designated in the will. Generally, executors are paid for administering the will, which can amount to considerable work, depending on the size and complexity of the estate. Typically, executors receive 3 to 4 percent of the total assets as payment for their service. If all goes well, a will is usually fully implemented within about one year of the individual's death.

To be confident that your assets are transferred as you wish, we suggest that you write a last will and testament—whether on your own, using one of the various forms or templates available on the Internet, or through a lawyer—and have your doctor make a note in your medical record that you were of sound mind when you made the will. Having this documentation in your medical chart may help avoid questions of your competence in writing the will should disagreements arise about entitlements and distribution of assets. Some people even videotape themselves reading their will so that visual and auditory evidence exists of their competency. A will can be changed at any time, and it should generally be updated if you have a substantial change in assets, if you change your mind about who to will your assets to, or if you move to another state.

When a will is contested, it is generally for one of two reasons. A potential beneficiary or other party may question whether the will is genuine and not a forgery, which underscores the critical need to have a will properly documented and witnessed. Someone may also claim that the deceased was not competent at the time of signing the version of the will in question and that a prior version is the true will to be executed.

In addition to indicating in a will how your property and assets should be distributed, it's a good idea to specify your preferences about cremation, burial, burial location, and a funeral or other memorial service. Giving as many details as possible will help family members immensely at such a difficult time.

High inheritance tax rates can be avoided by distributing money while still alive through gifts, trusts, and other avenues. As of this writing, anyone can donate up to $13,000 per year to individuals, churches, or charitable organizations without incurring federal estate tax or income tax.

■ ■ ■

If You Are Concerned about Making Your Wishes Known

- Plan ahead by researching long-term care options and making both advance directives and a last will and testament.
- Consult a lawyer to ensure that your advance directives and last will and testament cannot be misconstrued, that everything is properly documented and witnessed, and that documentation exists to confirm that you were clearly of sound mind at the time you signed the documents.
- Consider recording your wishes on an audiotape or videotape that would be played after your death.
- Keep copies of your advance directives and will in one or more safe places.
- Ask your doctor to keep a copy of your advance directives in your medical records.
- Organize all your financial records where they can be found easily.
- Give some thought to how you would like support care provided should you ever need it.
- Discuss your decisions and preferences with family members and trusted friends.

A Word about Elder Abuse: Suggestions for Family Members and Caregivers

Family members and caregivers should be aware of and on the lookout for elder abuse, a regrettable reality that may be perpetrated by hired caregivers, nursing home personnel, anonymous scam artists with fraudulent schemes, or the individual's own children. There are several forms of elder abuse:

- Physical abuse, which may be noticed by marks on the body such as bruises, welts, or burns. Unexplained injuries can also

indicate abuse, as can the use of inappropriate restraints. Sometimes an individual may witness inappropriate physical contact
or force being used on an older person.

- Emotional abuse, which may be occurring if an older person hesitates to talk or is evasive about a particular person or
situation. The older person may be withdrawn, anxious, or
depressed. Emotional abuse may also be indicated by different
people providing contradictory statements, or someone witnessing verbal hostility toward an older person.
- Neglect, which can include not ensuring that an older person
receives adequate nutrition and personal care. Forced isolation
and lack of follow-up medical care are also forms of neglect.
- Financial abuse or exploitation, which may be revealed by
withdrawals of assets from bank accounts, mounting credit
card charges, large "gifts" from the older person to another
individual, unpaid utility bills by a caregiver in charge of the
person's finances, or refusal to spend money on the older person
for necessary medical care, medications, dental care, or nursing home placement. Suspicion may be warranted if an older
person's will is reissued with a change in the recipients of the
estate shortly before the person dies or during a time when the
person was clearly demented or otherwise unable to use sound
judgment. Last, scams via mail, phone, and Internet or e-mail
frequently target older people. A person who responds to one of
these scams may then begin to receive frequent offers from scam
artists "competing" with each other for the person's money.
- Sexual abuse, which can be indicated by injuries to sexual
organs or by an older person contracting a new sexually transmitted infection. Older individuals may also report sexual abuse
themselves.

Many older people who become victims of abuse may not report
the abuse because of cognitive impairment or fear of reprisal. They
may also be embarrassed or think that they won't be believed. Doctors are required by law to report suspected abuse of elders to the
local Adult Protective Services agency, to track offenses and seek pro-
tection for vulnerable individuals. As a family member, a good way

to investigate suspected abuse at a care facility is to make frequent unannounced visits. Family members should also be alert for scams. If concerned, they can investigate setting up safeguards, such as joint bank accounts or agreements with a vulnerable elder to review or monitor assets and financial statements.

TWELVE

Finding Meaning and Fulfillment— and Fun

As people get older, they naturally tend to look back and try to make sense of how their life has unfolded, all the relationships they have had along their life's journey, and what they've done—and not done—during their lives. Taking time to search for personal meaning in one's life and celebrate the positive and memorable aspects can go far in helping to reduce anxiety and any tendency toward developing depression. Ideally, people will look back at their achievements and find a way to put them into a perspective that is meaningful and sustaining.

In this chapter, we discuss some ideas about finding satisfaction with your life's accomplishments, as well as continuing to live a fulfilling and rewarding life in your older years.

Reviewing and Accepting Your Life Accomplishments

Many people who struggle with anxiety or depression worry about their lives nearing the end and feel unfulfilled by their lives' work or activities. Some people feel a sense of not having accomplished what they had hoped to, while others worry about their children and grandchildren and wonder if they could have done more for them.

People use various ways to search for meaning and purpose as they look back over their lifetime. Religion and spirituality can be extremely important for many people, while others may look for books that discuss a philosophical approach to thinking about one's life. In addition, numerous memoirs, biographies, movies, and plays draw on the theme of finding meaning in life. These can be interesting for people who want to find out how others have viewed life and death.

Working on a family genealogy often proves to be absorbing and helps many people accept their place and contribution in their family's history. Writing, making audio or video recordings, or collaborating with an interested family member to help document an autobiography or memoir can be a wonderful way to record life events while also creating a treasure for younger generations in the family. Some people find that they can use writing or other means to tell stories that they have difficulty telling in person but that they feel are important stories to relate.

Reminiscing with other people can foster a sense of well-being about a particular accomplishment or simply provide validation for having survived a difficult time. A form of psychotherapy called *reminiscence therapy* encourages a group of people of similar age to listen to music, watch movies, or peruse photographs, newspapers, or magazines from a time earlier in their lives in order to evoke memories and exchange thoughts and feelings with each other. This type of reminiscence exercise might revolve around a particular theme for a couple of hours.

Perhaps the most difficult task for any reflective person is to come to terms with the inevitability of her death. Philosophers, religious leaders, and even scientists have all struggled with this issue, and there is plenty to read for people who like to take a scholarly approach. Ultimately, one's personal view counts the most. During moments of reflection, many people ask themselves some of these questions about life's meaning:

1. Why did my life turn out the way it did?
2. How do I fit in with the larger picture?
3. Have I lived my life well? What have I accomplished? What do I regret?
4. What do I feel I still need to do before I die?
5. How do I know if I can bear the final phase of my life if I die in some form of debilitation?
6. What legacy will I leave?
7. Whom do I worry about leaving behind after I'm gone?
8. What are my beliefs about what happens after I die?
9. Would I ever consider taking steps to end my life prematurely?

10. Have I told the people I care about most how much they mean to me?

For people who feel they have made their peace with one or more of these questions, a sense of meaning, purpose, or gratitude can deepen. Of course, some people may feel no need to even consider finding responses to these questions and are content to simply let the cards fall where they may. Some people are content to live in the moment without much reflection or forward thinking. There is no right or wrong way to think about these issues.

Finding Fulfillment in Your Older Years

Being "older" and thinking back on life in no way means that life is "over." On the contrary, older people can and do make significant contributions and find fulfillment. As always, different people take different approaches. Some of our patients describe simply being grateful for their lives continuing as they are and with all they contain; others focus their activities on "giving back" because they feel so much was given to them during their lives; and still others fulfill an inner need to keep learning new things.

Sometimes, however, the struggle with depression or anxiety worsens or becomes all-consuming as physical ailments limit a person's activities. We encourage people to take advantage of what is available at a given moment. For example, if someone has been very ill but now enjoys a period of better health, we encourage her to do something she had been putting off, such as taking a trip or visiting loved ones. Likewise, we suggest that people who struggle daily with pain, which is often accompanied by depression or anxiety, try to embrace small pleasures or diversions, such as visiting or phoning a friend, eating favorite foods, receiving a grandchild's artwork, taking a trip to a public garden, or just going for a drive in the countryside. Such small pleasures can be a counterbalance to life's everyday struggles and make the difference between enduring and embracing the day.

> Gloria was 73 when she first went to see a psychiatrist about depression, which was linked to her chronic pain in several arthritic joints and the consequent restrictions to her activities. She had tried all sorts

of pain remedies in combination with various antidepressants but had not found adequate relief. She admitted to the psychiatrist that she hoped he had something new to offer her. After reviewing her history, however, he told her that there were no unturned stones nor any quick fixes for her chronic pain.

The psychiatrist asked Gloria to describe her daily routine. She said she mostly stayed home watching TV. She complained that her pain was too severe to venture out much. The doctor told Gloria that her pain would likely never go away completely, no matter what pain remedy she used, and that she would do well to learn to live with it as best she could. Gloria was shocked to hear her doctor make this statement, and she simply stared at him. He continued by saying that she needed to decide whether she wanted to go somewhere and be in pain or merely stay at home and be in pain. If you go out, he said, you might find some diversion from your preoccupation with pain, but if you stay home, you'll never know what you might have missed and enjoyed. The doctor finished the conversation by saying that the choice was Gloria's, and he would be curious to hear what she decided to do.

Gloria left the office looking puzzled and quiet. She returned for a follow-up visit a month later to report that she had always wanted to make soup for one of her neighbors, an older man who lived alone. She proudly announced that she had actually done so, and the doctor complimented her on her initiative. During follow-up visits over the next several months, Gloria said that she was working on an art project with one of her grandchildren, and she went on to say that she was making plans to visit her other grandchildren, who didn't live nearby.

Gloria and her psychiatrist continued to talk about the theme of "what can you still do despite your pain?" and eventually Gloria stopped asking whether there were any new medications to try. Increasing her activity and enhancing her quality of life despite intractable pain and the accompanying feelings of demoralization and depression shifted her frame of mind. She had been putting her life on hold while waiting for complete relief from her pain, but now she was choosing to pursue activities that were important to her and that she could still manage despite her pain.

Successful aging involves adapting to life's circumstances using whatever resources are available. These resources might include practicing religion or spirituality, volunteering, being socially active, or maintaining family relationships. Research has shown that having an affiliation with a religious community can be protective against becoming depressed. Religious institutions can offer social support, a feeling of belonging, and a forum for spiritual renewal and guidance. There are also various spiritual fulfillments that are not easily categorized into an organized religion. For example, some people find fulfillment through reading or writing poetry, attending theater productions, learning about history, or listening to or playing music, to name only a few. Many people find solace in the beauty and wonder of nature and take time to immerse themselves regularly in natural environments. Some people find volunteering for charities and other organizations to be emotionally fulfilling, especially after retiring from a busy work life. Participating in these types of activities can help people find meaning, structure, guidance, and a sense of purpose.

Having social connections can become critical as people age. Being socially active, whether with a few close friends and family members or with larger groups of people through clubs and organizations, can help combat loneliness, demoralization, and depression. Most people will need some sort of assistance at some point, so having a network of friends and family to rely on for emotional or practical support at these times can really help. The reciprocal is also true: people who participate in a social network may find opportunities to help another person in need as well. People who successfully return to leading a fulfilling life after their spouse passes away typically have sought out companionship. Cultivating new friendships can be hard, especially when moving to live in a new location, but it isn't impossible. Phone calls and e-mail can help maintain connections to old friends, while joining a group, taking a class, or participating in activities at a recreation or seniors' center can lead to making new friends.

Family relationships can be a complex mixture of shared joy, gratitude, duty, and history—both good and bad. Relationships may be caring and of great comfort, but they might also produce conflict and anxiety. Perhaps because of changing roles over time, adult children and their parents sometimes have difficulty finding the right balance for being involved in each others' lives without being intrusive on the one hand or neglectful on the other. Disputes can cause distress, which can lead to anxiety and depression. Fortunately, in many instances, grandchildren are a balm that makes visiting and regular interaction pleasant no matter what tensions still exist between the adult children and parents.

Counseling or psychotherapy may help people involved in a difficult relationship to see the problem from different points of view, place past psychological wounds in a new perspective, and find new strategies for meaningful communication. Psychotherapy can feel liberating and validating, even if the other person in a difficult relationship doesn't appear ready for compromise. Research has shown that maintenance psychotherapy, even just monthly, can keep anxiety low and prevent future episodes of depression by helping people recall and reinforce improved coping strategies they learned in psychotherapy.

A Healthy Body for a Healthy Mind

Frequently in this book, we've mentioned the positive benefits of staying physically healthy to promote and maintain mental health. Good health habits, such as getting adequate rest, eating a balanced diet, getting regular exercise, and cutting back or avoiding alcohol, caffeine, and nicotine, can stabilize biological rhythms and help ensure good mental health for the long term. The body and mind truly are connected.

We believe that living as an older adult without the added burden of depression or excessive anxiety is an achievable goal worth pursuing by everyone, and we sincerely hope that some or all of the chapters in this book have provided a measure of insight and guidance toward achieving that goal.

ACKNOWLEDGMENTS

We would like to acknowledge the following individuals who offered editorial review and advice: Mary Ganguli, M.D., Frank Costa, M.D., Mark Musmano, M.D., Eric Rodriguez, M.D., Ann Germain, Ph.D., Daniel Buysse, M.D., Lin Ehrenpreis, L.C.S.W., Antoine Douihay, M.D., Howard Kline Esq., and Jordan Karp, M.D.

We would particularly like to thank Eric M. Miller, B.S., for his extensive editing and research assistance.

General
Aging
AARP (formerly the American Association of Retired Persons,
    www.aarp.org
ElderCare Online, www.ec-online.net
U.S. Administration on Aging, www.aoa.gov

Medical
Mayo Clinic, www.mayoclinic.com
WebMD, www.webmd.com

Suicide Prevention
National Hopeline Network, www.hopeline.com, 1-800-SUICIDE
    (784-2433)
National Suicide Prevention Lifeline, www.suicidepreventionlifeline.org,
    1-800-273-TALK (8255)

Support
HelpGuide.org, www.helpguide.org

Chapter 1. What You Need to Know about Depression
Further Reading

Bellenier, K., editor. 2009. *Mental Health Disorders Sourcebook*. 4th edition.
    Detroit, Mich.: Omnigraphics.
Berlin, E. 1998. *The Blues: Not a Normal Part of Aging*. San Francisco:
    American Society on Aging. Video recording.
Ellison, J. M., and H. H. Kyomen. 2009. *Mood Disorders in Later Life*. 2nd
    edition. New York: Informa Healthcare.
Erickson, E. H. 1980. *Identity and the Life Cycle*. New York: Norton.

Golant, M., and S. K. Golant. 2007. *What to Do When Someone You Love Is Depressed: A Practical, Compassionate and Helpful Guide.* New York: Henry Holt.

Judd, S. J., editor. 2008. *Depression Sourcebook.* 2nd edition. Detroit, Mich.: Omnigraphics.

Katon, W. 2008. *The Depression Helpbook.* Boulder, Colo.: Bull Publishing.

Lake, J. H., and D. Spiegel, editors. 2007. *Complementary and Alternative Treatments in Mental Health Care.* 1st edition. Washington, D.C.: American Psychiatric Publishing.

Miller, M. D., and C. F. Reynolds III. 2002. *Living Longer Depression Free: A Family Guide to Recognizing, Treating, and Preventing Depression in Later Life.* Baltimore, Md.: Johns Hopkins University Press.

Mischoulon D., and J. F. Rosenbaum. 2002. *Natural Medications for Psychiatric Disorders: Considering the Alternatives.* Philadelphia: Lippincott Williams & Wilkins.

Mondimore, F. M. 2006. *Bipolar Disorder: A Guide for Patients and Families.* 2nd edition. Baltimore, Md.: Johns Hopkins University Press.

Mondimore, F. M. 2006. *Depression, the Mood Disease.* 3rd edition. Baltimore, Md.: Johns Hopkins University Press.

Moyers, B. 1993. *Healing and the Mind.* New York: Doubleday.

Shorter, E. 2007. *Shock Therapy: A History of Electroconvulsive Treatment in Mental Illness.* New Brunswick, N.J.: Rutgers University Press.

Wulsin, L. R. 2007. *Treating the Aching Heart: A Guide to Depression, Stress, and Heart Disease.* Nashville, Tenn.: Vanderbilt University Press.

Zarit, S. H., and B. G. Knight. 1996. *A Guide to Psychotherapy and Aging: Effective Clinical Interventions in a Late-Stage Context.* 1st edition. Washington, D.C.: American Psychological Association.

Support and Information

Depression and Bipolar Support Alliance (DBSA), www.dbsalliance.org

Mental Health America (formerly the National Mental Health Association), www.nmha.org

National Alliance on Mental Illness, www.nami.org

National Mental Health Consumers' Self-Help Clearinghouse, http://mhselfhelp.org

Chapter 2. What You Need to Know about Anxiety
Further Reading

Rabins, P. V., and L. Lauber. 2005. *Getting Old without Getting Anxious: Conquering Late-Life Anxiety.* New York: Avery.

Support and Information

Anxiety Disorders Association of America, www.adaa.org

National Panic and Anxiety Disorder News, www.npadnews.com

Chapter 3. Coping with Memory Loss
Further Reading

Cohen, D., and C. Eisdorfer. 2001. *The Loss of Self: A Family Resource for the Care of Alzheimer's Disease and Related Disorders*. Revised and updated edition. New York: Norton.

Mace, N. L., and P. V. Rabins. 2011. *The 36-Hour Day: A Family Guide to Caring for People Who Have Alzheimer Disease, Related Dementias, and Memory Loss*. 5th edition. Baltimore, Md.: Johns Hopkins University Press.

Shenk, D. 2001. *The Forgetting: Alzheimer's, Portrait of an Epidemic*. New York: Anchor Books.

Support and Information

Alzheimer's Association, www.alz.org

Alzheimer's Foundation of America, www.alzfdn.org

Chapter 4. Living with Illness and Disability
Further Reading

Goldstein, M. S. 1999. *Alternative Health Care: Medicine, Miracle or Mirage?* Philadelphia: Temple University Press.

Lieberman, A. 2002. *Parkinson Disease: Fighting Like a Tiger, Thinking Like a Fox*. Sudbury, Mass.: Jones and Bartlett Publishers.

Servan-Schreiber, D. 2004. *The Instinct to Heal: Curing Stress, Anxiety, and Depression without Drugs and without Talk Therapy*. Emmaus, Pa.: Rodale.

Servan-Schreiber, D. 2009. *Anticancer: A New Way of Life*. New York: Viking.

Shannon, J. B., editor. 2008. *Disease Management Sourcebook*. 1st edition. Detroit, Mich.: Omnigraphics.

Steptoe, A., editor. 2007. *Depression and Physical Illness*. Cambridge: Cambridge University Press.

Sutton, A. L., editor. 2008. *Stroke Sourcebook*. 2nd edition. Detroit, Mich.: Omnigraphics.

Support and Information

American Association of People with Disabilities, www.aapd.com

American Diabetes Association, www.diabetes.org

American Heart Association, www.heart.org
American Stroke Association, www.strokeassociation.org
Arthritis Foundation, www.arthritis.org
National Stroke Association, www.stroke.org

Chapter 5. Getting Relief from Physical Pain
Further Reading

Information Television Network. 2006. *Chronic Pain*. New York: Films for the Humanities & Sciences. Video recording.
Jay, G. W. 2007. *Chronic Pain*. New York: Informa Healthcare.
Marcus, D. 2009. *Chronic Pain*. 2nd edition. New York: Humana Press.
Ranjan, R. R. 2006. *Chronic Pain and Family: A Clinical Perspective*. New York: Springer.

Support and Information

American Pain Foundation, www.painfoundation.org
National Pain Foundation, www.nationalpainfoundation.org

Chapter 6. Understanding Sleep and Fatigue
Further Reading

Judd, S. J., editor. 2010. *Sleep Disorders Sourcebook*. 3rd edition. Detroit, Mich.: Omnigraphics.
Wilson, V. A. 1996. *Sleep Thief, Restless Legs Syndrome*. Orange Park, Fla.: Galaxy Books.

Support and Information

American Sleep Association, www.sleepassociation.org
National Sleep Foundation, www.sleepfoundation.org

Chapter 7. Coping with the Loss of a Loved One
Further Reading

Didion, J. 2005. *The Year of Magical Thinking*. New York: Knopf.
Tatelbaum, J. 1980. *The Courage to Grieve: Creative Living, Recovery, and Growth through Grief*. New York: Harper & Row.

Support and Information

Good Grief Center, www.goodgriefcenter.com
HelpGuide.org, www.helpguide.org/mental/grief_loss.htm

Chapter 8. Stopping Overuse of Alcohol or Prescription Drugs
Further Reading

Atkinson, R. M. 1984. *Alcohol and Drug Abuse in Old Age*. Washington,
D.C.: American Psychiatric Press.

Beechem, M. H. 2002. *Elderly Alcoholism: Intervention Strategies*. Springfield,
Ill.: Charles C Thomas.

Support and Information

Al-Anon, www.al-anon.alateen.org
Alcoholics Anonymous, www.aa.org
Nar-Anon, www.nar-anon.org
Narcotics Anonymous, www.na.org
National Institute on Alcohol Abuse and Alcoholism, www.niaaa.nih.gov

Chapter 9. Maintaining Healthy Body Weight and Nutrition
Further Reading

Kessler, D. 2009. *The End of Overeating: Taking Control of the Insatiable North
American Appetite*. Emmaus, Pa.: Rodale.

Rolfes, S. R. 2009. *Understanding Normal and Clinical Nutrition*. Belmont,
Calif.: Wadsworth/Cengage Learning.

Support and Information

ChooseMyPlate.gov, U.S. Department of Agriculture, www.choosemyplate
.gov
Dietary Guidelines for Americans 2010, U.S. Department of Agriculture,
www.choosemyplate.gov/dietary-guidelines.html
Sit and Be Fit: A Non-Profit Organization Committed to Healthy Aging,
www.sitandbefit.org
Weight-Control Information Network, U.S. Department of Health and
Human Services and the National Institutes of Health, http://win.niddk
.nih.gov/publications/physical.htm

Chapter 10. Preserving (or Renewing) Sexual Pleasure
Further Reading

Hanash, K. A. 2008. *New Frontiers in Men's Sexual Health: Understanding
Erectile Dysfunction and the Revolutionary New Treatments*. Westport,
Conn.: Praeger Publishers.

Roszler, J., and D. Rice. 2007. *Sex and Diabetes: For Him and for Her*. Alex-
andria, Va.: American Diabetes Association.

Wingert, P., and B. Kantrowitz. 2006. *Is It Hot in Here? Or Is It Me?: The Complete Guide to Menopause*. New York: Workman.

Support and Information
Mayo Clinic, www.mayoclinic.com (search for "Sexuality" on the home page)
Sexual Health, www.sexualhealth.com

Chapter 11. Planning for Life's Final Phase
Further Reading
Dolan, S. R., and A. Vizzard. 2009. *The End of Life Advisor: Personal, Legal, and Medical Considerations for a Peaceful, Dignified Death*. New York: Kaplan.

Feldman, D. B. 2007. *The End-of-Life Handbook: A Compassionate Guide to Connecting with and Caring for a Dying Loved One*. Oakland, Calif.: New Harbinger Publications.

Kuebler, K. K., D. E. Heidrich, and P. Esper. 2007. *Palliative and End-of-Life Care: Clinical Practice Guidelines*. 2nd edition. Philadelphia: Saunders.

Satterfield, J. M. 2008. *A Cognitive-Behavioral Approach to the Beginning of the End of Life: Minding the Body: Facilitator Guide*. Oxford: Oxford University Press.

Silverstone, B., and H. K. Hyman. 2008. *You and Your Aging Parent: A Family Guide to Emotional, Social, Health, and Financial Problems*. 4th edition. Oxford: Oxford University Press.

Support and Information
Assisted Living Federation of America, www.alfa.org
Caring Connections: National Hospice and Palliative Care Organization, www.caringinfo.org
Five Wishes document, www.agingwithdignity.org/five-wishes.php
Hospice Foundation of America, www.hospicefoundation.org
U.S. Administration on Aging, www.aoa.gov

Chapter 12. Finding Meaning and Fulfillment—and Fun
Further Reading
Rowe, J. W., and R. L. Kahn. 1998. *Successful Aging*. New York: Pantheon Books.

Shield, R. R. 2003. *Aging in Today's World: Conversations between an Anthropologist and a Physician*. New York: Berghahn Books.

SELECTED REFERENCES

Preface

Dominus, S. 2004. Life in the age of old, old age. *New York Times Magazine*, February 2, pp. 26–60.

Reichstadt, J., C. A. Depp, L. A. Palinkas, et al. 2007. Building blocks of successful aging: A focus group study of older adults' perceived contributors to successful aging. *American Journal of Geriatric Psychiatry* 15(3):194–201.

Sakauye, K. 2008. *Geriatric Psychiatry Basics*. 1st edition. New York: Norton.

Spar, J. E., and A. La Rue. 2005. *Concise Guide to Geriatric Psychiatry*. 2nd edition. Washington, D.C.: American Psychiatric Press.

Chapter 1. What You Need to Know about Depression

American Psychiatric Association. 2000. *Diagnostic and Statistical Manual of Mental Disorders*. 4th edition, text revised. Washington, D.C.: American Psychiatric Association.

Brenner, R., L. Bjerkenstedt, and G. V. Edman. 2002. *Hypericum perforatum* extract (St. John's wort) for depression. *Psychiatric Annals* 32(1):21–26.

Brown, R. P., and P. L. Gerbarg. 2001. Herbs and nutrients in the treatment of depression, anxiety, insomnia, migraine, and obesity. *Journal of Psychiatric Practice* 7:75–91.

Bruce, M. L., T. R. Ten Have, C. F. Reynolds, et al. 2004. Reducing suicidal ideation and depressive symptoms in depressed older primary care patients: A randomized controlled trial. *Journal of the American Medical Association* 291(9):1081–91.

Consumer Health Digest. 2011. Omega-3 Fatty Acids and Depression. www.consumerhealthdigest.com/omegafattyacids.htm.

Conwell, Y. 1994. Suicide in elderly patients. In *Diagnosis and Treatment of Depression in Late Life*, edited by L. S. Schneider, C. F. Reynolds, and

B. D. Lebowitz, 397–418. Washington, D.C.: American Psychiatric Press.

Demitrack, M. A. 2007. Therapeutic neuromodulation: Clinical and research implications of a new therapeutic platform. *Psychiatric Annals* 37(3):165–74.

Dunner, D. L. 2003. Treatment considerations for depression in the elderly. *CNS Spectrums* 8(12 suppl. 3):14–19.

Engels, G., and M. Vermey. 1997. Efficacy of nonmedical treatments of depression in elders: A quantitative analysis. *Journal of Clinical Geropsychology* 31:17–35.

Frank, E. 2005. *Treating Bipolar Disorder: A Clinician's Guide to Interpersonal and Social Rhythm Therapy*. Guides to Individualized Evidence-Based Treatment. 1st edition. New York: Guilford Press.

George, L. K. 2004. Social and economic factors related to psychiatric disorders in late life. In *The American Psychiatric Publishing Textbook of Geriatric Psychiatry*, edited by D. G. Blazer, D. C. Steffens, and E. W. Busse, 139–61. Washington, D.C.: American Psychiatric Press.

Heisel, M. J. 2006. Suicide and its prevention among older adults. *Canadian Journal of Psychiatry* 51(3):143–54.

Husain, M. M., A. J. Rush, H. A. Sackeim, et al. 2005. Age-related characteristics of depression: A preliminary STAR*D report. *American Journal of Geriatric Psychiatry* 13(10):852–60.

Kales, H. C., D. F. Maixner, and A. M. Mellow. 2005. Cerebrovascular disease and late-life depression. *American Journal of Geriatric Psychiatry* 13(2):88–98.

Karel, M. J., and G. Hinrichsen. 2000. Treatment of depression in late life: Psychotherapeutic interventions. *Clinical Psychology Review* 20(6):707–29.

Kramer, P. D. 2005. *Against Depression*. New York: Viking Penguin.

Kyomen, H. H., and T. H. Whitfield. 2009. Psychosis in the elderly. *American Journal of Psychiatry* 166(2):146–50.

Linden, D. E. L. 2006. How psychotherapy changes the brain—the contribution of functional neuroimaging. *Molecular Psychiatry* 11(6):528–38.

Mast, B. T., A. R. Azar, and S. A. Murrell. 2005. The vascular depression hypothesis: The influence of age on the relationship between cerebrovascular risk factors and depressive symptoms in community dwelling elders. *Aging and Mental Health* 9(2):146–52.

Miller, M. D., C. Cornes, E. Frank, et al. 2001. Interpersonal psychotherapy for late-life depression: Past, present, and future. *Journal of Psychotherapy Practical Research* 10(4):231–38.

Millon, T. 1995. *Disorders of Personality: DSM-IV and Beyond*. New York: Wiley-Interscience.

National Institute of Mental Health. 2008. *Mental Health Medications*. NIH Publication No. 08-3929. Revised.

Pies, R. 2000. Adverse neuropsychiatric reactions to herbal and over-the-counter "antidepressants." *Journal of Clinical Psychiatry* 61(11):815–20.

Pinquart, M., and S. Sorensen. 2001. How effective are psychotherapeutic and other psychosocial interventions with older adults? *Journal of Mental Health and Aging* 7:207–43.

Reynolds, C. F., E. Frank, J. M. Perel, et al. 1999. Nortriptyline and interpersonal psychotherapy as maintenance therapies for recurrent major depression: A randomized controlled trial in patients older than 59 years. *Journal of the American Medical Association* 281(1):39–45.

Richelson, R. 2007. Mechanisms of action of repetitive Transcranial Magnetic Stimulation (rTMS) and Vagus Nerve Stimulation (VNS). *Psychiatric Annals* 37(3):181–87.

Rush, A. J., J. Kilner, M. Fava, et al. 2008. Clinically relevant findings from STAR*D. *Psychiatric Annals* 38(3):188–93.

Schulberg, H. C., E. P. Post, P. J. Raue, et al. 2007. Treating late-life depression with interpersonal psychotherapy in the primary care sector. *International Journal of Geriatric Psychiatry* 22(2):106–14.

Schulz, R., S. R. Beach, R. S. Hebert, et al. 2009. Spousal suffering and partner's depression and cardiovascular disease: The Cardiovascular Health Study. *American Journal of Geriatric Psychiatry* 17(3):246–54.

Scogin, F., D. Welsh, A. Hanson, et al. 2005. Evidence-based psychotherapies for depression in older adults. *Clinical Psychology of Science Practices* 12:222–37.

Shea, M. T. 1993. Personality disorders and depression: An overview of issues and findings. *Rhode Island Medicine* 76(8):405–8.

Sternbach, H. 2003. Psychiatric manifestations of low testosterone in men. *Psychiatric Annals* 33(8):517–24.

Szanto, K., H. G. Prigerson, and C. F. Reynolds. 2001. Suicide in the elderly. *Clinical Neuroscience Research* 1:366–76.

Teri, L., and S. McCurry. 2000. Psychosocial therapies. In *American Psychiatric Press Textbook of Geriatric Neuropsychiatry*, edited by C. E. Coffey and J. L. Cummings, 861–90. Washington, D.C.: American Psychiatric Press.

Vataja, R., T. Pohjasvaara, R. Mantyla, et al. 2005. Depression-executive dysfunction syndrome in stroke patients. *American Journal of Geriatric Psychiatry* 13(2):99–107.

Waern, M., E. Rubenowitz, B. Runeson, et al. 2002. Burden of illness and suicide in elderly people: Case-control study. *British Medical Journal* 324(7350):1355.

Chapter 2. What You Need to Know about Anxiety

Beaudreau, S. A., and R. O'Hara. 2008. Late-life anxiety and cognitive impairment: A review. *American Journal of Geriatric Psychiatry* 16(10):790–803.

Bisson, J. I., M. Brayne, F. M. Ochberg, et al. 2007. Early psychosocial intervention following traumatic events. *American Journal of Psychiatry* 164(7):1016–19.

Chou, K. L. 2009. Age at onset of generalized anxiety disorder in older adults. *American Journal of Geriatric Psychiatry* 17(6):455–64.

Food and Drug Administration. 2007. *Caffeine in My Home: Caffeine and Your Body*. Publication UCM205286.pdf, www.fda.gov.

Healthwise. 2008. Medicines That Can Cause Anxiety. www.revolution health.com/conditions/mental-behavioral-health/anxiety/causes/medications-cause-anxiety.

Jeste, N. D., J. C. Hays, and D. C. Steffens. 2006. Clinical correlates of anxious depression among elderly patients with depression. *Journal of Affective Disorders* 90(1):37–41.

Mayo Foundation for Medical Education and Research. 2009. Caffeine Content for Coffee, Tea, Soda and More. www.mayoclinic.com/health/caffeine/AN01211.

Mischoulon, D. 2002. The herbal anxiolytics kava and valerian for anxiety and insomnia. *Psychiatric Annals* 32(1):55–60.

Schoevers, R. A., D. J. H. Deeg, W. van Tilburg, et al. 2005. Depression and generalized anxiety disorder: Co-occurrence and longitudinal patterns in elderly patients. *American Journal of Geriatric Psychiatry* 13(1):31–39.

Chapter 3. Coping with Memory Loss

American Psychiatric Association. 2000. *Diagnostic and Statistical Manual of Mental Disorders*. 4th edition, text revised. Washington, D.C.: American Psychiatric Association.

Cummings, J. L. 2004. Dementia with Lewy bodies: Molecular pathogenesis and implications for classification. *Journal of Geriatric Psychiatry and Neurology* 17(3):112–19.

Dolder, C. R. 2004. Diagnosis and treatment of psychiatric and behavioral disturbances in Alzheimer disease: A review of recent literature. *Current Psychosis and Therapeutics Reports* 2(1):13–20.

Elliott, R. 2003. Executive functions and their disorders. *British Medical Bulletin* 65(1): 49–59.

Ellison, J. M. 2008. Mild cognitive impairment. *CNS Spectrums* 13(1):41–42.

Goveas, J. S., M. Dixon-Holbrook, D. Kerwin, et al. 2008. Mild cognitive impairment: How can you be sure? *Current Psychiatry* 7(4):37–50.

Hashimoto, M., H. Kazui, K. Matsumoto, et al. 2005. Does donepezil treatment slow the progression of hippocampal atrophy in patients with Alzheimer's disease? *American Journal of Psychiatry* 162(4):676–82.

Hughes, T. F., and M. Ganguli. 2009. Modifiable risk factors for late-life cognitive impairment and dementia. *Current Psychiatry Reviews* 5:73–92.

Kiosses, D. N., and G. S. Alexopoulos. 2005. IADL functions, cognitive deficits, and severity of depression: A preliminary study. *American Journal of Geriatric Psychiatry* 13(3):244–49.

Lantz, M. S. 2009. Who cares for the caregiver? *Clinical Geriatrics* 17(10): 6–8.

Lee, H. B., and C. G. Lyketsos. 2004. Diagnosis and clinical management of depression in mild cognitive impairment. *Psychiatric Annals* 34(4):273–80.

Li, I., and R. V. Smith. 2003. Driving and the elderly. *Clinical Geriatrics* 11(5):40–46.

McGuire, L. C., E. S. Ford, and U. A. Ajani. 2006. Cognitive functioning as a predictor of functional disability in later life. *American Journal of Geriatric Psychiatry* 14(1):36–42.

Miller, M. D. 1989. Opportunities for psychotherapy in the management of dementia. *Journal of Geriatric Psychiatry and Neurology* 2(1):11–17.

Miller, M. D. 2009. *Clinician's Guide to Interpersonal Psychotherapy in Late Life: Helping Cognitively Impaired or Depressed Elders and Their Caregivers.* Oxford: Oxford University Press.

Miller, M. D., V. Richards, A. Zuckoff, et al. 2006. A model for modifying interpersonal psychotherapy (IPT) for depressed elders with cognitive impairment. *Clinical Gerontologist* 302(2):79–101.

Parks, S. M., and K. D. Novielli. 2003. Alzheimer's disease caregivers: Hidden patients. *Clinical Geriatrics* 11(5):34–38.

Pollock, B. G., B. H. Mulsant, J. Rosen, et al. 2007. A double-blind comparison of citalopram and risperidone for the treatment of behavioral and psychotic symptoms associated with dementia. *American Journal of Geriatric Psychiatry* 15(11):942–52.

Ritchie, C. W., D. Ames, T. Clayton, et al. 2004. Metaanalysis of randomized trials of the efficacy and safety of donepezil, galantamine, and rivastigmine for the treatment of Alzheimer disease. *American Journal of Geriatric Psychiatry* 12(4):358–69.

Ropacki, S. A., and D. V. Jeste. 2005. Epidemiology of and risk factors for psychosis of Alzheimer's disease: A review of 55 studies published from 1990 to 2003. *American Journal of Psychiatry* 162(11):2022–30.

Rosenberg, P. B., D. Johnston, and C. G. Lyketsos. 2006. A clinical approach to mild cognitive impairment. *American Journal of Psychiatry* 163(11):1884–90.

Ross, R. 1993. The pathogenesis of atherosclerosis: A perspective for the 1990s. *Nature* 362(6423):801–9.

Sano, M. 2003. Current concepts in the prevention of Alzheimer's disease. *CNS Spectrum* 8(11):846–53.

Spar, J. E., and A. LaRue. 2006. Other dementias and delirium. In *Clinical Manual of Geriatric Psychiatry*, 229–72. Washington, D.C.: American Psychiatric Publishing.

Tune, L. E. 2004. Anticholinergic delirium: Assessing the role of anticholinergic burden in the elderly. *Current Psychosis and Therapeutics Reports* 2(1):33–36.

Twin Cities Public Television. 2004. *The Forgetting: A Portrait of Alzheimer's*. St. Paul, Minn.: Twin Cities Public Television.

Valenzuela, M., and P. Sachdev. 2009. Can cognitive exercise prevent the onset of dementia? Systematic review of randomized clinical trials with longitudinal follow-up. *American Journal of Geriatric Psychiatry* 17(3):179–87.

Wagner, A. W., R. G. Longsdon, J. L. Pearson, et al. 1997. Caregiver expressed emotion and depression in Alzheimer's disease. *Aging and Mental Health* 1(2):132–39.

Yurchenko, A., M. I. Lapid, and K. A. Josephs. 2009. Frontotemporal dementia in older adults: Diagnostic and therapeutic challenges. *Clinical Geriatrics* 17(1):26–31.

Chapter 4. Living with Illness and Disability

Bremmer, M. A., W. J. Hoogendijk, D. J. Deeg, et al. 2006. Depression in older age is a risk factor for first ischemic cardiac events. *American Journal of Geriatric Psychiatry* 14(6):523–30.

De Ronchi, D., F. Bellini, D. Berardi, et al. 2005. Cognitive status, depressive symptoms, and health status as predictors of functional disability among elderly persons with low-to-moderate education: The Faenza Community Aging Study. *American Journal of Geriatric Psychiatry* 13(8):672–85.

Lyness, J. M., E. D. Caine, Y. Conwell, et al. 1993. Depressive symptoms, medical illness, and functional status in depressed psychiatric inpatients. *American Journal of Psychiatry* 150(6):910–15.

McEwen, B. S. 2008. Central effects of stress hormones in health and disease: Understanding the protective and damaging effects of stress and stress mediators. *European Journal of Pharmacology* 583(2–3):174–85.

Newton, T. L., and J. M. Sanford. 2003. Conflict structure moderates associations between cardiovascular reactivity and negative marital interaction. *Health Psychology* 22(3):270–78.

Rovner, B. W., R. J. Casten, and B. E. Leiby. 2009. Variability in depressive symptoms predicts cognitive decline in age-related macular degeneration. *American Journal of Geriatric Psychiatry* 17(7):574–81.

Schulberg, H. C., R. Schulz, M. D. Miller, et al. 2000. Depression and physical illness in older primary care patients: Diagnostic and treatment issues. In *Physical Illness and Depression in Older Adults: A Handbook of Theory, Research, and Practice*, edited by G. M. Williamson, D. R. Shaffer, and P. A. Parmelee, 239–56. New York: Kluwer Academic / Plenum Publishers.

Sussman, J., and S. Altman. 2009. How will we meet the health services needs of an aging America? Policy Brief from the 16th Princeton Conference, sponsored by the Council on Health Care Economics and Policy, May 20–21.

Turvey, C. L., S. K. Schultz, L. Beglinger, et al. 2009. A longitudinal community-based study of chronic illness, cognitive and physical function, and depression. *American Journal of Geriatric Psychiatry* 17(8):632–41.

WebMD. Drugs That Cause Depression. 2005. www.webmd.com/depression/guide/medicines-cause-depression.

Wheaton, J., and S. M. Pinkstaff. 2006. Atherosclerotic vascular disease and diabetes in the older adult. Part I: Understanding pathogenic mechanisms and identifying risk factors. *Clinical Geriatrics* 14(1):17–23.

Chapter 5. Getting Relief from Physical Pain

Freeman, R. 2009. The treatment of neuropathic pain. *CNS Spectrum* 10(9):698–706.

Leveille, S. G., R. N. Jones, D. K. Kiely, et al. 2009. Chronic musculoskeletal pain and the occurrence of falls in an older population. *Journal of the American Medical Association* 302(20):2214.

Vastag, B. 2003. Scientists find connections in the brain between physical and emotional pain. *Journal of the American Medical Association* 290(18):2389–90.

Weiner, D. K. 2010. Pain in Older Adults. http://nationalpainfoundation.org/articles/162/pain-in-older-adults.

Chapter 6. Understanding Sleep and Fatigue

Baron, K. G., T. W. Smith, L. A. Czajkowski, et al. 2009. Relationship quality and CPAP adherence in patients with obstructive sleep apnea. *Behavioral Sleep Medicine* 7(1):22–36.

Benca, R. M., M. Okawa, M. Uchiyama, et al. 1997. Sleep and mood disorders. *Sleep Medicine Reviews* 1(1):45–56.

Edinger, J. D., and W. S. Sampson. 2003. A primary care "friendly" cognitive behavioral insomnia therapy. *Sleep* 26, 177–82.

Fetveit, A. 2009. Late-life insomnia: A review. *Geriatrics and Gerontology International* 9(3):220–34.

Geriatric Mental Health Foundation. 2008. *Sleeping Well as We Age.* Bethesda, Md.: Geriatric Mental Health Foundation.

Germain, A., D. E. Moul, P. L. Franzen, et al. 2006. Effects of a brief behavioral treatment for late-life insomnia: Preliminary findings. *Journal of Clinical Sleep Medicine* 2:403–6.

Morin, C. M. 2004. Cognitive-behavioral approaches to the treatment of insomnia. *Journal of Clinical Psychiatry* 65 (suppl. 16):33–40.

Ramakrishnan, K., and D. C. Scheid. 2007. Treatment options for insomnia. *American Family Physician* 76(4):517–26.

Reid, K. J., Z. Martinovich, S. Finkel, et al. 2006. Sleep: A marker of physical and mental health in the elderly. *American Journal of Geriatric Psychiatry* 14(10):860–66.

Reishtein, J. L., A. I. Pack, G. Maislin, et al. 2006. Sleepiness and relationships in obstructive sleep apnea. *Issues in Mental Health Nursing* 27(3):319–30.

Walsh, J. K. 2004. Pharmacologic management of insomnia. *Journal of Clinical Psychiatry* 65(suppl. 16):40–45.

Chapter 7. Coping with the Loss of a Loved One

Engel, G. L. 1961. Is grief a disease? A challenge for medical research. *Psychosomatic Medicine* 23(1):18–22.

Miller, M. D., E. Frank, C. Cornes, et al. 1994. Applying interpersonal psychotherapy to bereavement-related depression following loss of a spouse in late life. *Journal of Psychotherapy Practice and Research* 3(2):149–62.

Schulz, R. 2005. Effects of bereavement on family members: Examining the evidence of Alzheimer's disease caregivers. *ElderCare* 5(3):1–2.

Shear, M. K., E. Frank, P. R. Houck, et al. 2005. Treatment of complicated grief: A randomized controlled trial. *Journal of the American Medical Association* 293(21):2601–8.

Simon, N. M., M. K. Shear, E. H. Thompson, et al. 2007. The prevalence and correlates of psychiatric comorbidity in individuals with complicated grief. *Comprehensive Psychiatry* 48(5):395–99.

Chapter 8. Stopping Overuse of Alcohol or Prescription Drugs

About.com. Medical Treatments for Alcoholism. http://alcoholism.about .com/od/meds/Medical_Treatments_for_Alcoholism.htm. Accessed September 15, 2011.

Alcoholics Anonymous. 1976. *The Story of How Many Thousands of Men and Women Have Recovered from Alcoholism.* 3rd edition. New York: Alcoholics Anonymous World Services.

Alcoholism in the Population. www.alcoholism-statistics.com/facts.php. Accessed November 30, 2011.

Anda, R. F., D. F. Williamson, L. G. Escobedo, et al. 1990. Depression and the dynamics of smoking: A national perspective. *Journal of the American Medical Association* 264(12):1541–45.

Anstey, K. J., H. A. Mack, and N. Cherbuin. 2009. Alcohol consumption as a risk factor for dementia and cognitive decline: Meta-analysis of prospective studies. *American Journal of Geriatric Psychiatry* 17(7):542–55.

Association Against Steroid Abuse. "Dangers of Steroid Abuse." www .steroidabuse.com/dangers-of-steroid-abuse.html. Accessed June 24, 2011.

Centers for Disease Control and Prevention (CDC). 2011. Health Effects of Cigarette Smoking. www.cdc.gov/tobacco/data_statistics/fact_sheets/ health_effects/effects_cig_smoking/index.htm.

Ewing, J. A. 1984. Detecting alcoholism: The CAGE questionnaire. *Journal of the American Medical Association* 252:1905–7.

Mathews, S., and D. W. Oslin. 2009. Alcohol misuse among the elderly: An opportunity for prevention. *American Journal of Psychiatry* 166(10):1093–95.

Moos, R. H., K. K. Schutte, et al. 2009. Older adults' alcohol consumption and late-life drinking problems: A 20-year perspective. *Addiction* 104:1293–1302.

National Institute on Drug Abuse. Prescription Drug Abuse Chart. www .nida.nih.gov/drugpages/prescripdrugschart.html. Accessed June 24, 2011.

U.S. Department of Agriculture and U.S. Department of Health and Human Services. 2010. *Dietary Guidelines for Americans, 2010.* Washington, D.C.: Government Printing Office.

U.S. Department of Health and Human Services. 2001. *Women and Smok-*

ing: A Report of the Surgeon General. Rockville, Md.: U.S. Department of Health and Human Services, Public Health Service, Office of the Surgeon General.

Winkel, V., and B. Bair. 2008. Substance use disorders in older adults. *Clinical Geriatrics* 16(7):25–29.

World Health Organization. 2001. *The Alcohol Use Disorders Identification Test: Guidelines for Use in Primary Care—Audit*. 2nd edition. Geneva: World Health Organization.

Chapter 9. Maintaining Healthy Body Weight and Nutrition

Centers for Disease Control and Prevention (CDC). 2011. Physical Activity for Everyone. www.cdc.gov/physicalactivity/everyone/health.

Kessler, D. A. 2009. *The End of Overeating*. Emmaus, Pa.: Rodale.

U.S. Department of Agriculture. 2011. Dietary Guidelines for Americans 2010, www.choosemyplate.gov/dietary-guidelines.html.

Chapter 10. Preserving (or Renewing) Sexual Pleasure

Basson, R. 2008. Women's sexual function and dysfunction: Current uncertainties, future directions. *International Journal of Impotence Research* 20(5):466–78.

Brecher, E. M. 1984. *Love, Sex and Aging*. Boston: Little, Brown.

Ginsberg, T. B., and T. A. Cavalieri. 2008. Androgen deficiency in the aging male: The beginning, the middle, and the ongoing. *Clinical Geriatrics* 16(4):25–28.

Hodson, D. S., and P. Skeen. 1994. Sexuality and aging: The hammerlock of myths. *Journal of Applied Gerontology* 13:219–35.

Chapter 11. Planning for Life's Final Phase

Cooper, C., A. Selwood, and G. Livingston. 2009. Knowledge, detection, and reporting of abuse by health and social care professionals: A systematic review. *American Journal of Geriatric Psychiatry* 17(10):826–38.

FindLaw.com. 2008. "FindLaw Survey: Most Americans Don't Have a Will." http://commonlaw.findlaw.com/2008/06/findlaw-survey.html.

Genworth Financial. 2011. Genworth 2011 Cost of Care Survey: Home Care Providers, Adult Day Health Care Facilities, Assisted Living Facilities and Nursing Homes. www.genworth.com/content/products/long_term_care/long_term_care/cost_of_care.html.

Lantz, M. S. 2004. Elder abuse: Making a difference. *Clinical Geriatrics* 12(12):37–40.

Lewis, M. A., and K. S. Rook. 1999. Social control in personal relationships: Impact on health behaviors and psychological distress. *Health Psychology* 18(1):63–71.

Lo, B., D. Ruston, L. W. Kates, et al. 2002. Discussing religious and spiritual issues at the end of life: A practical guide for physicians. *Journal of the American Medical Association* 287(6):749–54.

Rook, K. S., P. D. Thuras, and M. A. Lewis. 1990. Social control, health risk taking, and psychological distress among the elderly. *Psychology and Aging* 5(3):327–34.

U.S. Administration on Aging. National Clearinghouse for Long-Term Care Information. Costs of Care. www.longtermcare.gov/LTC/Main_Site/Paying/Costs/Index.aspx. Accessed November 30, 2011.

Chapter 12. Finding Meaning and Fulfillment—and Fun

Hebert, R. S., Q. Dang, and R. Schulz. 2007. Religious beliefs and practices are associated with better mental health in family caregivers of patients with dementia: Findings from the REACH study. *American Journal of Geriatric Psychiatry* 15(4):292–300.

Koenig, H. G. 2007. Religion and depression in older medical inpatients. *American Journal of Geriatric Psychiatry* 15(4):282–91.

Lantz, M. S. 2007. Religion and coping in late life. *Clinical Geriatrics* 15(8):16–19.

Sbarra, D. A. 2009. Marriage protects men from clinically meaningful elevations in C-reactive protein: Results from the National Social Life, Health, and Aging Project (NSHAP). *Psychosomatic Medicine* 71(8):82.

Page numbers in *italics* indicate tables.